Basic Decompression Theory And Application

B.R. Wienke

88-70554
Library of Congress Catalog Card Number
ISBN 0-941332-17-9
International Standard Book Number

PRINTED AND BOUND IN THE UNITED STATES

BEST PUBLISHING COMPANY
2355 North Steves Boulevard
P.O. Box 30100
Flagstaff, AZ 86004
USA

ABSTRACT

The monograph discusses working decompression models in fundamental theory and application. Classical dissolved gas models are detailed first, followed by more recent phase models. Specific model issues are presented, along with the rationale behind dive tables and meters. Decompression statistics and risk analysis are also treated. Bounce, repetitive, multiday, decompression, and saturation exposures are contrasted within the models. Emphasis is placed on phase dynamical considerations. Mathematical developments are summarized in Appendices. Some prior knowledge of decompression theory is helpful, but not requisite for this monograph.

Pages — 105, Figures — 19, Tables — 10, Appendices — 6

Keywords — Decompression Theory, Mathematical Models, Phase Dynamics, Bubbles And Nucleation, Tables

AUTHOR SKETCH

Bruce Wienke is a Section Head in the Applied Theoretical Physics Division of the Los Alamos National Laboratory, located in New Mexico, with interests in computational decompression and models, gas transport, and phase mechanics. He is an Instructor Trainer with the National Association Of Underwater Instructors (NAUI), serving on the Decompression Review Board, a Master Instructor with the Professional Association Of Diving Instructors (PADI), serving on the Instructor Review Committee, and an Institute Director with the YMCA. He also works as a ski racing coach and instructor, functioning as clinician with the United States Ski Coaches Association (USSCA) and the Professional Ski Instructors of America (PSIA). Bruce received a MS in nuclear physics from Marquette University, and a PhD in particle physics from Northwestern University. He works closely with the American Physical Society, American Nuclear Society, Society Of Industrial And Applied Mathematics, Undersea And Hyperbaric Medical Society, and the American Academy Of Underwater Sciences, serving as a Fellow and Technical Committee Member in various capacities. Bruce is also the author of the monograph, "High Altitude Diving".

TABLE OF CONTENTS

LIST OF TABLES

LIST OF FIGURES

PREFACE

This exposition attempts to walk a line between a discussion of decompression theory with equations and corresponding dialogue using extended prose. Both theory and diving application are, at times, more an artform than exact science. Some physiologists take the view that deterministic modeling can only be fortuitous. Technological advance, elucidation of competing mechanisms, and resolution of model issues over the past 80 years has not been rapid. Model applications tend to be *ad hoc,* tied to data fits, and difficult to quantify on first principles. Almost any description of decompression processes in tissue and blood can be disputed, and possibly turned around on itself. The fact that decompression sickness occurs in metabolic and perfused matter makes it difficult to design and analyze experiments outside living matter. Yet, for application to safe diving, we need models to build tables and meters. And deterministic models, not discounting shortcomings, are the real subject of this monograph.

The reader will notice an emphasis on free gas phases (bubbles, nuclei, and whatever else is not dissolved), and comments about free phase models versus (just) dissolved phase models, the present basis for most decompression analysis. Most of the comments are based on recent experiments coupled to basic physics. While we do not know all the facts yet, the author takes the view that phase models correlated with available data, linked to underlying physical principles, and which recover dissolved gas models in appropriate limits, are the types of models which should be extended, refined, and used in table and meter algorithms. The alternative to model algorithms is statistical analyses of decompression risk data, folded into meaningful and useful meter format, an area under active study by US Navy investigators and others.

The intent here is to present a working view of decompression in diving, mostly focusing on theory with application, and without tedious equations which are reserved for the Appendices in more than casual analysis. The discussion is neither a medical nor physiological synthesis. Such aspects are simplified, and for some certainly oversimplified. Nonetheless, it is directed toward the diver and reader with some rudimentary understanding of decompression. A background in the physical or life sciences is helpful, but certainly not requisite. Only the basic mechanisms of tissue gas exchange, bubbles and nucleation, supersaturation, perfusion and diffusion, and related topics are discussed. The Appendices draw only on rudimentary calculus, and only to qualify discussion. To be general and concise is to be careful of trying not to cover too much ground. And that is the tack here. In the same vein, discussion is limited to Type I and II bends, limb and central nervous system hits, not Type III and IV, vestibular dysfunction and bone necrosis. The primary insult in the former cases is thought to be bubbles, while in the latter cases other factors come more into play.

The organization of the monograph is simple. Roughly, the first half discusses dissolved gas models and the second half describes free phase models which incorporate dissolved gas models as subsets. Issues and applications are presented for both. Operational procedures for tables and meters are also outlined. Discussion is necessarily limited to inert nitrogen decompression in air mixtures, though results in many cases extend to other mixtures. A statistical approach to decompression, essentially model independent, is also described. Appendices outline some of the mathematical equations and assumptions implicit to models. References, neither exhaustive nor necessarily elementary, but representative of the lore, are also included.

Many thanks to colleagues and friends for their interest, including Tom Kunkle (LANL), David Yount (University of Hawaii), Charles Lehner and Ed Lanphier (University of Wisconsin), Gerry Pomraning (UCLA), and Paul Weathersby (NSMRL), as well as diving organizations, including the National Association of Underwater Instructors (NAUI), the Professional Association of Diving Instructors (PADI), and the YMCA. Special thanks to the Los Alamos National Laboratory (LANL) for personal support. Affiliations with the American Academy Of Underwater Sciences (AAUS) and the Undersea And Hyperbaric Medical Society (UHMS) have also been informative and helpful, as well as the American Physical Society (APS), the American Nuclear Society (ANS), and the Society of Industrial And Applied Mathematics (SIAM). Thanks go to the Professional Ski Instructors Of America (PSIA) and the United States Ski Coaches Association (USSCA) for a casual reading of the manuscript. Finally, SCUBAPRO Industries has been very supportive of modeling work for meter implementations, and special thanks to Richard Bonin, Jim Dexter, and Doug Toth for their help and interest.

Standard units are employed mainly in development. However, by convention, because of literature usage, or for convenience, some non-standard units are also used. Such units have become a part of the diving lore. For instance, pressures and depths are both quoted in feet-of-sea-water *(fsw)*, with 1 *atm* = 33 *fsw.* A unit of length, called the *micron,* is also convenient with 1 *micron* = 10^{-4}*cm.* Frequency is defined in *megahertz,* with 1 *megahertz* = 10^{6} *cycles/sec.* Atomic weight is given in *atomic mass* units *(amu),* for 1 *amu* = 1.66 x 10^{-24}*g.* Elevation in altitude is measured conveniently in feet *(ft).*

This monograph is dedicated to my wife and diving partner, Cynthia. Her interest and enthusiasm will always be appreciated.

CHAPTER 1

Background

Increases in pressure with increasing depth underwater impose many of the limitations in diving, applying equally well to the design of equipment used in this environment. Early divers relied on their breathholding ability, while later divers used diving bells. Surface supplied air and SCUBA are rather recent innovations. With increasing depth and exposure time, divers encountered a number of physiological and medical problems constraining activity, with decompression sickness perhaps the more restrictive. By the 1800s, bubbles were noted in animals subject to pressure reduction. In the 1900s, they were postulated as the cause of decompression sickness in caisson workers and divers. Within that postulate, and driven by a need to both optimize diver safety and time underwater, decompression modeling has consolidated early rudimentary schedules into present more sophisticated tables. As knowledge and understanding of decompression sickness increase, so should the validity, reliability, and range of applicability models.

1.1 HISTORY

Breathhold diving dates as far back as Xerxes and Alexander the Great, according to the Greek historian Herodotus, and reed breathing tubes were employed by the Roman Legions. Primitive diving bells also date BC, though the inverted receptacles employing Boyle's law of compressed air as breathing mixture gained renown in the 1600s. Persians also carried air in goatskins underwater. Today, Korean and Japanese breathhold divers still gather pearls and sponges in the old way.

Surface supplied air and demand regulators were employed in hard hat diving by the 1800s, with the first demand regulator, patented by Rouquayrol in 1866, supplied by hand-operated bellows. The first case of nitrogen narcosis was reported by Junod in 1835. Full suits, in which air escapes through a one way exhaust valve, were invented in 1840, and some are still in use. Quietly, the revolutionary *aqua lung* of Cousteau, a refinement of the Rouquayrol surface supplied demand regulator, ushered the modern era of SCUBA in wartime Europe in 1943. Diving was never the same afterward. Freed from any surface umbilical, the Cousteau unit revolutionized underwater warfare to be sure, but the impact on non-military diving was an order of magnitude greater. Coupled to high pressure compressed air in tanks, SCUBA offered the means to explore the underwater world for fun and profit.

Commercial availability of the demand regulator in 1947 initiated sport diving, and a fledgling equipment industry. Serious diver training and certifying agencies, such as the YMCA and National Association of Underwater Instructors, organized in the late 1950s and 1960s. In the mid 1950s, the Royal Navy (RN) released their bulk diffusion decompression tables, while a little later, in 1958, the US Navy (USN) compiled their modified Haldane tables with six perfusion limited compartments. Both would acquire biblical status over the next 25 years, or so. In the mid to late 1950s, Fredrickson in the USA and Alinari in Italy designed and released the first analog decompression meters, emulating tissue gas uptake and elimination with pressure gauges, porous plugs, and distensible gas bags. The first digital computers, designed by DCIEM in Canada, appeared by the mid 1950s. Employed by the Canadian Navy, they were based on the earlier four compartment analog model of Kidd and Stubbs. Following introduction of a twelve compartment Haldanian device, correlated with Doppler measurements by Barshinger and Huggins in 1983, decompression computers reached a point of maturation and acceptance. Flexible, more reliable, easier to use, and able to emulate almost any mathematical model, digital computers rapidly replaced pneumatic devices in the 1980s. Their timely functionality and widespread use heralded the present era of hi-tech diving, with requirements for comprehensive decompression models across a full spectrum of activity.

Diver mobility concerns ultimately fostered development of the modern SCUBA unit, and the quest to go deeper led to exotic gas breathing mixtures. High pressure cylinders and compressors similarly expedited deeper diving and prolonged exposure time. The world record dives of Keller to 1000 *fsw* in 1960 not only popularized multiple gas mixtures, but also witnessed first use of computers to generate decompression schedules. Saturation diving and underwater habitats followed soon after, spurred by a world thirst for oil. Both multiple gas mixtures and saturation diving became a way of life for some commercial divers by the 1970s, particularly after the oil embargo.

Cochrane in England invented the high pressure caisson in 1830. Shortly afterward, the first use of a caisson in 1841 in France by Triger also witnessed the first case of decompression sickness, properly termed the bends because of the position assumed by victims to alleviate the pain. Some fifty eight years later, in 1889, the first medical lock was employed by Moir to treat the bends during construction of the Hudson River tunnel. Since that time many divers and caisson workers have been treated in hyperbaric chambers. Indeed, the operational requirements of diving over the years have provided the incentives to study hyperbaric physiology and its relationship to decompression sickness, as well as the impetus for biophysical models.

1.2 GAS TRANSFER AND PHYSIOLOGY

The pulmonary and circulatory systems are connected gas transfer networks. Lung blood absorbs oxygen from inspired air in the alveoli, and releases carbon dioxide into the alveoli. The surface area for exchange in the lungs is enormous, on the order of a few hundred $meters^2$. Nearly constant values of alveolar partial pressures of oxygen and carbon dioxide are maintained by the respiratory centers, with ventilated alveolar volume near 4 *liters* in adults. The partial pressure of inspired oxygen is usually higher than the partial presssure of tissue and blood oxygen, and the partial pressure of inspired carbon dioxide less, balancing metabolic requirements of the body.

Gas usually moves in direction of decreased concentration in any otherwise homogeneous medium with uniform solubility. If there exist regions of varying solubility, this is not necessarily true. For instance, in the body there are at least two tissue types, one predominantly aqueous (watery) and the other lipid (fatty), varying in solubility by a factor of five for nitrogen. That is, nitrogen is five times more soluble in lipid tissue than aqueous tissue. If aqueous and lipid tissue are in nitrogen equilibrium, then a gaseous phase exists in equilibrium with both. Both solutions are said to have a nitrogen *tension* equal to the partial pressure of the nitrogen in the gaseous phase. The concentration of the dissolved gas in each species equals the product of the solubility times the tension, according to Henry's law. If two nitrogen solutions, one lipid and the other aqueous, are placed in contact, nitrogen will diffuse towards the solution with decreased nitrogen tension. The driving force for the transfer of any gas is the pressure gradient, whatever the phases involved, liquid-to-liquid or gas-to-liquid. Tension and partial pressure have the same dimensions. The volume of gas that diffuses under any gradient is a function of the interface area, solubility of the media, and distance transversed. The rate at which a gas diffuses is inversely proportional to the square root of its atomic weight. Following equalization, dissolved volumes of gases depend upon their individual solubilities in the media.

The circulatory system, consisting of the heart, arteries, veins, and lymphatics, convects blood throughout the body. Arterial blood leaves the left heart via the aorta (2.5 *cm*), with successive branching of arteries until it reaches arterioles (30 *microns*), and then systemic capillaries (8 *microns*) in peripheral tissues. These capillaries join to form venules (20 *microns*), which in turn connect with the vena cava (3 *cm*), which enters the right heart. During return, venous blood velocities increase from 0.5 *cm/sec* to nearly 20 *cm/sec.* Blood leaves the right heart through the pulmonary arteries on its way to the lungs. Following oxygenation in the lungs, blood returns to the left heart through the pulmonary veins, beginning renewed arterial circulation.

Blood has distinct components to accomplish many functions. Plasma is the liquid part, carrying nutrients, dissolved gases (excepting oxygen), and some chemicals, and makes up some 55% of blood by weight. Red blood cells (erythrocytes) carry the other 45% by weight, and through the protein hemoglobin, transport oxygen to the tissues. Enzymes in red blood cells also participate in a chemical reaction transforming carbon dioxide to a bicarbonate in blood plasma. The average adult carries about 5 *liters* of blood, 30-35% in the arterial circulation (pulmonary veins, left heart, and systemic circulation), and 65-70% in the venous flow (veins and right heart). About 9.5 *ml* of nitrogen are transported in each *liter* of blood. Arterial and venous tensions of metabolic gases, such as oxygen and carbon dioxide, differ, while blood and tissue tensions of water vapor and nitrogen are the same. Arterial oxygen tensions exceed venous tensions, while venous carbon dioxide tensions exceed arterial tensions. Oxygen tissue tensions are below both arterial and venous tensions, while carbon dioxide tissue tensions exceed both. Arterial tensions equilibrate with alveolar (inspired air) partial pressures in less than a minute. Such an arrangement of tensions in the tissues and circulatory system provides the necessary pressure head between alveolar capillaries of the lungs and systemic capillaries pervading extracellular tissue space.

Tissues (and venous blood) are typically unsaturated with respect to inspired air (and arterial tension) somewhere in the vicinity of 8-13% of ambient pressure. That is, summing up partial pressures of inspired gases in air, total venous and tissue tensions fall short in that percentage range. Carbon dioxide produced by metabolic processes is twenty-five times more soluble than oxygen consumed, and hence exerts a lower partial pressure by Henry's law. This tissue debt is called the *inherent unsaturation,* or *oxygen window* in diving applications.

1.3 DECOMPRESSION SYNDROME

Decompression sickness results from excessive changes in ambient pressure over a particular period of time. In simple decompression sickness, Types I and II, bubbles, or some related form of free gas phase, are thought to trigger a complex chain of physico-chemical reactions in the body, affecting the pulmonary, neurological, and circulatory systems adversely. Treatment consists of recompression, usually in a hyperbaric chamber with controlled application of ambient pressure. Increasing ambient pressure tends to shrink the bubbles by Boyle's law, reducing size, and dissolve bubbles by increasing constrictive surface tension pressure, tending to collapse them. Strategic introduction of oxygen can also aid in the washing out of inert gases during decompression. Bubbles have been found in intravascular (arteries, veins, lymphatics) and extravascular (intracellular, extra-cellular) sites upon decompression. Many factors are relevant to the formation of bubbles, such as gas uptake and elimination in the tissues and blood, gas solubility and diffusivity, tissue vascularity and type, breathing mixture, amount of pressure reduction, temperature, presence of preformed nuclei, and individual susceptibility.

Decompression sickness is classified into four major categories, with the first two sometimes labeled simple decompression sickness. Of course, nothing is simple about decompression sickness. The categories are:

(1) Type I (limb bends); characterized by local pain in the extremities, itching, red spots, swelling, or muscle stiffness affecting the knees, elbows, hips, muscles, or skin;
(2) Type II (central nervous system bends); characterized by confusion, paralysis, pain in the chest, breathing difficulty, or unconsciousness affecting the brain, spinal cord, or lungs;
(3) Type III (vestibular bends); characterized by hearing impairment, vertigo, tinnitus (ringing and buzzing), or nausea occurring with exposures beyond the 300 *fsw* range affecting the balance organs of the ear; and
(4) Type IV (dysbaric osteonecrosis); characterized by bone lesions, structural damage, or local mineralization, occurring with repeated exposures to high pressure environments, affecting the long bones.

Type I and II are thought to be caused primarily by bubbles, and related ischemia (blood chemistry change). Type III may involve bubbles, inert gas counter-diffusion, and fluid shifts in the vestibular organs. Type IV remains more of a mystery, possibly bubbles, ischemia, emboli, and combinations of all. Rapid and repeated compression and carbon dioxide retention are also concerns in Type IV. Our concerns are bubbles and models in simple decompression sickness, Types I and II, a much narrower focus.

Bert first noted that when a group of subjects were decompressed together after the same exposure most would be unaffected, and only one might be afflicted with decompression sickness. Such differences are due both to the random nature of bubble formation and variations in individual tolerance to bubbles formed after every decompression. As discussed by Bennett and Elliott, individual susceptibilities depend on a number of factors:

(1) Age; generally the older the person, especially over 40, the greater the susceptibility to decompression sickness;
(2) Obesity; leaner subjects are less disposed to decompression sickness;
(3) Exercise; exercise during, and after, decompression is thought to increase the likelihood of decompression sickness, by increased gas uptake in the former case and agitation in the latter;
(4) Fluid Balance: dehydration is known to increase disposition to decompression sickness, and is physically linked to low surface tension of blood serum which does not inhibit bubble growth optimally;
(5) Alcohol; alcohol also reduces blood serum surface tension, increasing decompression sickness likelihood;
(6) Temperature; colder environmental temperatures are known to increase susceptibility to decompression sickness;
(7) Adaptation; progressively greater tolerance to the effects of decompression during a series of consecutive exposures has been demonstrated;
(8) Injuries; injury sites are more predisposed to bubble formation.

Knowledge of the pathology of the clinical manifestations of decompression sickness is incomplete today, yet some understanding of the nature of decompression sickness is fundamental to methods directed towards prevention and treatment. Symptoms of decompression sickness occur after reduction in ambient pressure, and relax following treatment by recompression, pointing to bubbles, seen by Boyle as early as 1670 in animals decompressing at altitude, as the culprit. Procedures for prevention and treatment are still based upon that premise, at least for Type I and II decompression sickness. Treatment is not the focus in the following, but rather prevention according to mathematical models, ostensibly translated into dive tables, decompression schedules, or meter algorithms.

In applying models to complex phenomena, like decompression sickness, frameworks are only as strong as the facts upon which they are built. With decompression sickness, facts are not superabundant. Conversely, some models can overlook the facts, in which case they lose predictive capability, reducing their utility. In any case, modelers are chartered with the ambivalent task of extracting the facts and invoking the proper physical models, knowing full well that the complement of assumptions is approximate.

1.4 HALDANE MODEL

Tables and schedules for diving at sea level can be traced to a model proposed in 1908 by the eminent English physiologist, John Scott Haldane. He observed that goats, saturated to depths of 165 feet-of-sea water *(fsw)* did not develop decompression sickness (DCS) if subsequent decompression was limited to half the ambient pressure. Extrapolating to humans, researchers reckoned that tissues tolerate elevated dissolved gas pressures (tensions), greater than ambient by factors of two, before the onset of symptoms. Haldane then constructed schedules which limited the critical supersaturation ratio to two in hypothetical tissue compartments. Tissue compartments were characterized by their half-life, τ, that is, the time required for the compartment to halve (lose) or double (gain) dissolved nitrogen. Five compartments (5, 10, 20, 40, 75 *minutes*) were employed in decompression calculations and staged procedures for fifty years. In performing deep diving and expanding table ranges in the 1930s, Hawkins and Shilling, and Yarborough, assigned separate limiting tensions (*M*-Value) to each tissue compartment. Later in the 1950s and early 1960s, Dwyer, Des Granges, and Workman, in addressing repetitive exposures for the first time, advocated the use of six tissues (5, 10, 20, 40, 80, 120 *minutes*) in constructing decompression schedules, with each tissue compartment again possessing its own limiting tension. Temporal uptake and elimination of inert gas was based on mechanics addressing only the macroscopic aspects of gas exchange between blood and tissue. Exact bubble production mechanisms, interplay of free and dissolved gas phases, and related transport phenomena were not quantified, since they were neither known nor understood. Today, we know much more about dissolved and free phase dynamics, bubbles, and transport mechanisms, but still rely heavily on the Haldane model. Inertia and simplicity tend to sustain its popularity and use, and it has been a workhorse.

Basically, the Haldane model is a dissolved gas approach, with the assumption that bubbles form *de novo* (spontaneously) in supersaturated tissue under decompression. Such mechanism appears possible under explosive (very rapid) decompression, but less so in controlled situations. To spontaneously form bubbles in fluids under explosive decompression requires pressure reductions near 1000 *atm*, stressing fluids to their so-called tensile limits, certainly outside nominal diving range. Similarly, recent experiments suggest the existence of preformed, and very small, seed pockets of gas in tissues, growth-excitable under decompression. Additionally, chemists tell us that spontaneous bubble formation thresholds are ill-defined in heterogeneous media, like tissue, and that critical tensions are metastable (variation range is infinite over small range of initial conditions). Adding this all up, many regard the Haldane model as a useful fit to the data, appropriate to bounce diving, yet more limited as proportions of free gas phases grow under repetitive loading.

CHAPTER 2

Dissolved Gas Phase Models

Dissolved gas models limit degrees of tissue supersaturation, assuming gas exchange is controlled by perfusion (blood flow rate) or gaseous diffusion in blood-tissue media. Exchange of inert gas is driven by the local *gradient,* that is, the difference between the arterial blood and local tissue tension. Obviously the exchange process is very complicated, and models are only approximate. Consider the perfusion limited exchange model first. Historically, it emerged early in the Boycott and Damant studies of decompression and dominated models for many years, as charted in the work of Behnke, Hawkins and Schilling, Yarborough, Dwyer, Des Granges, Buhlmann, and Workman.

2.1 PERFUSION MODEL

Perfusion limited gas exchange is modeled in time by mathematical classes of *exponential* response functions, bounded by arterial and initial tissue tensions, described in Appendix A. Compartments with 1, 2.5, 5, 10, 20, 40, 80, 120, 240, 360, and 720 minute half-lives, τ, are employed in applications today, and half-lives are assumed to be independent of pressure. A one-to-one correspondence between compartments and specific anatomic entities is neither established, nor implied. For large values of τ, tissue uptake and elimination of inert gas is relatively slow according to the response function. For small values of τ, inert gas uptake and elimination proceed much more rapidly. According to Kety, and Kety and Schmidt, the major controlling factor is the blood flow rate, $1/\tau$ effectively. Actually, gas uptake and elimination in all tissues is not controlled just by perfusion. Diffusion may dominate in certain tissue types, regions with lesser vascularity and greater distance between capillaries, such as bone and spinal cord. In others, both perfusion and diffusion are rate limiting. Modeling tissue gas exchange is not a simple process, particularly since we know little about tissue compositions in any type of decompression sickness, and even less of tissue sites.

The rate of uptake and elimination of inert gas is assumed to be symmetric when the same set of tissue half-lives are employed in calculations. However, this is not always the case. Microbubbles in the circulatory system, particularly venous gas emboli, render gas uptake and elimination asymmetric. Bubbles in the interstitial areas, or agglutination of red blood cells in reaction to foreign bubbles would have similar effect on local perfusion rates. In such instances, half-lives for uptake are then shorter than half-lives for elimination.

To maximize uptake or elimination of inspired gases, the gradient should be maximized. Maximization of this gradient, however, must never permit dissolved gas buildup above critical limits for each compartment, and hence the requirement for staging ascents when tensions exceed critical limits. Haldane theory limits degrees of absolute compartment supersaturation by critical values, M, having a modern range, $122 \leq M \leq 36$ *fsw*, notably of American origin. In bubble theories, supersaturation is limited by the relative difference, or critical gradient, G, between the absolute tissue tension and ambient partial pressure, that is, $G = M/.79 - P$, for P the ambient pressure. The factor .79 converts the nitrogen critical tensions to absolute pressure units. In decompressed gel experiments, Strauss suggested that $G \approx 20$ *fsw,* for pressures less than a few atmospheres. Other studies suggest, $10 \leq G \leq 30$ *fsw*, as a range of critical gradients (G-Values).

Early studies employed fixed values for M and G, but today critical parameters generally vary across compartments, and with depth. Supersaturation theories regard the critical parameters as trigger points for bubble formation, while bubble theories might view the critical parameters as signal points for clinical manifestation of symptoms, following bubble growth to damaging size. Bubble criteria, G, are more fundamental than tension criteria, M, but Haldane limiting tensions enjoy widespread popularity. Historically, the critical ratios, R (critical tensions divided by ambient pressure, or R-values) were first employed in analyses. Quite obviously, R and M are equivalent sets, differing only by a multiplicative factor P, the ambient pressure.

2.2 CRITICAL TENSIONS

Critical parameters evolved from self-consistent application of assumed tissue response to sets of exposure data, that is, trial and error bootstrapping of model equations to observed exposure time limits. Newer compilations ultimately extend older ones in like manner, as described by Schreiner and Hamilton. The critical tensions suggested by Workman and Buhlmann for arbitrary compartments are well known, and, along with the previously mentioned exponential tissue function, are the esential elements of the Haldane approach. Surfacing critical tensions M_0, surfacing critical ratios, R_0, at sea level, and changes per foot depth, ΔM, are listed in Table 1 under appropriate headings. At depth, d, the critical tension is the sum of M_0 and ΔMd, that is, $M = M_0 + \Delta Md$. Critical tensions and ratios are also plotted in Figures 1a and 1b, all according to Workman (USN). Such parameters form the basis for most tables and meter algorithms, with a noted recent tendency to reduce critical tensions and non-stop bounce time limits for safety sake. In the case of single tissue diffusion models, a single set of equivalent parameters is employed in like manner.

Table 1. Surfacing Ratios And Critical Tensions ($P_0 = 33$ *fsw*).

half-life τ *(minutes)*	**surface ratio** R_0	**surface tension** M_0 *(fsw)*	**tension change** ΔM
5	**3.15**	**104**	**2.27**
10	**2.67**	**88**	**2.01**
20	**2.18**	**72**	**1.67**
40	**1.76**	**58**	**1.34**
80	**1.58**	**52**	**1.26**
120	**1.55**	**51**	**1.19**

Blood rich, well-perfused, aqueous tissues are usually thought to be *fast* (small τ), while blood poorer, scarcely-perfused, lipid tissues are thought to be *slow* (large τ) though the spectrum of half-lives is not correlated with actual perfusion rates in critical tissues. As reflected in Table 1, critical parameters are obviously larger for faster tissues. The range of variation with compartment and depth is not small, as seen in Figure 1a. Surfacing values are principal concerns in dissolved gas staging regimens, dictated by the necessity to maximize gradients through upward excursion. Phase models focus on the amount of separated gas, with corresponding pressure balance requiring gradients for bubble elimination to *increase* with depth, directly opposite to dissolved gas elimination gradients which *decrease* with depth. Then decompression becomes a playoff between dissolved gas buildup and free phase growth, tempered by body ability to eliminate both. That playoff is a central issue in decompression modeling and staging procedures.

Figure 1a. Perfusion Limited Critical Tensions.

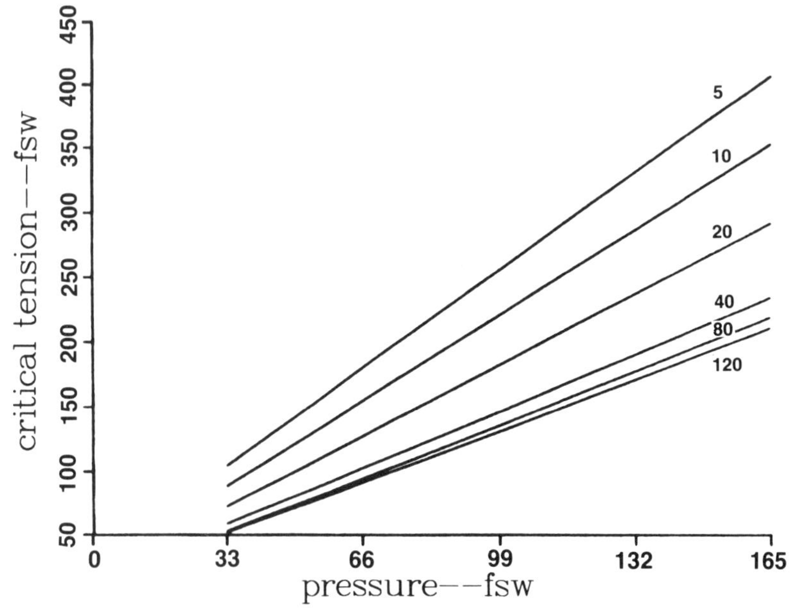

Critical tensions are fitted linear functions of pressure, obviously increasing with ambient pressure. Faster compartments permit greater amounts of dissolved nitrogen, slower compartments less. During any dive, tensions in compartments must stay below the depicted curves in this modified Haldane approach. Wienke reduced the USN critical tensions to an approximate form (fsw),

$$M = 152.7\tau^{-1/4} + 3.25\tau^{-1/4}\, d,$$

for depth d (fsw). Dividing critical tensions by ambient pressure, P, yields the critical ratios, R. Extensions of the curves to altitude (P < 33 fsw) have been effected linearily and exponentially. In the linear case, the zero pressure intercepts are positive, while in the exponential case the intercepts are zero. Thus, in the former case, critical ratios become unbounded at zero ambient pressure, while in the latter case, they remain finite. Any set of non-stop time limits can be plugged into model equations and ensuing sets of tensions for compartments can be scanned for maximum values across all depths and half-lives.

2.3 REDUCED ATMOSPHERIC PRESSURE

Decompression at reduced ambient pressure, $P < 33$ *fsw,* has been a study in itself, as reported by many such as Buhlmann, Boni and Schibli, Edel and Carroll, Bell and Borgwardt, Gray and Masland, Bassett, Lanphier, and Lehner, to mention just a few. Recent thinking is nicely summarized by Sheffield. Decompression studies developed separately above and below sea level, referenced as aerial and underwater decompression, also by the adjectives, hyperbaric and hypobaric.

Aerial decompression differs from routine underwater decompression because the blood and tissues are equilibrated (saturated) with nitrogen ambient pressure before ascent. Breathing pure oxygen before ascent helps

Figure 1b. Perfusion Limited Critical Ratios.

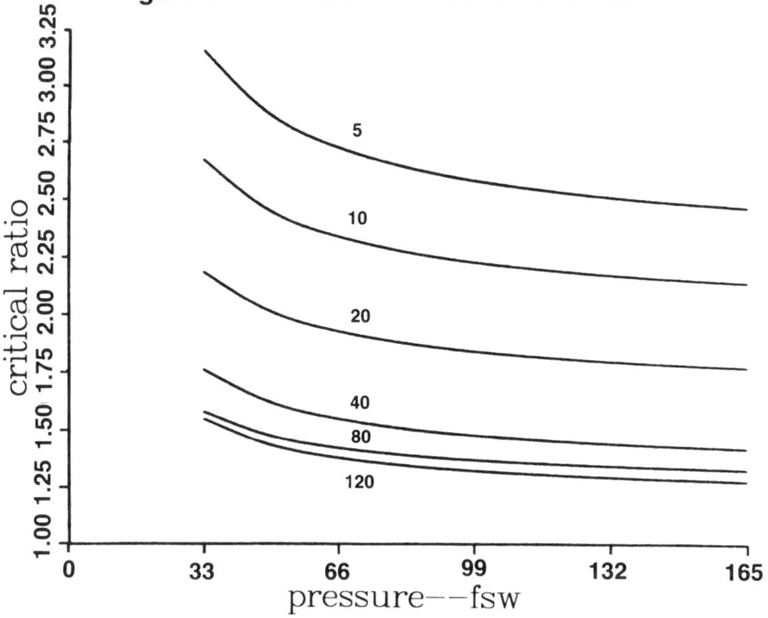

The critical ratios, R, are hyperbolic functions of pressure. For each of the six tissue compartments, the above ratios permit greater degrees of supersaturation in the faster compartments, as also witnessed by the critical tensions. If the critical tensions in Figure 1a are linearily extrapolated to altitude ($P \leq 33$ fsw), then the critical ratios approach infinity as the ambient pressure drops. However, if the critical tensions decrease exponentially with ambient pressure, the critical ratios remain finite and bounded. As seen in Figure 5, constant ratio, R, extrapolations are limited in scope of application, not applying to saturation diving and probably not to heavy multi-diving activities.

to protect against decompression sickness by washing out nitrogen. Up to about 18000 *ft*, such procedure offers a considerable degree of protection. Beyond that, according to Behnke, silent bubbles may retard nitrogen elimination. Simple bubble mechanics suggest that bubble excitation and growth are enhanced as ambient pressure decreases, and so decompression problems are theoretically exacerbated by altitude. Nucleation theory also suggests that critical radii increase with decreasing pressure, offering larger, less stable gas seeds for possible excitation and growth into bubbles. Larger bubbles possess smaller constricting surface tensions, and will thus grow faster in conducive situations. Such facts have been verified in the laboratory, and follow from simple bubble theory. Certainly the same considerations confront the diver at altitude, and are compounded with increasing nitrogen tension upon surfacing at reduced atmospheric pressure.

Lower pressures at elevation, and the lower density of fresh water to a lesser degree, affect gas uptake and elimination rates in tissues and blood. If critical tensions are employed to limit exposures, an immediate question centers upon their extrapolation and testing at altitude. Looking at Figure 1a, a linear extrapolation of the critical tensions seems obvious, indeed just such an extrapolation of the USN critical tensions was proposed and tested by Bell and Borgwardt. Buhlmann, employing a different set of half-lives and critical tensions, also extended the Haldane algorithm to altitudes near 10000 *ft*. Along with reduced critical tensions at altitude, reduced non-stop time limits, compared to sea level, are a natural consequence. Another approach reduces the critical tensions exponentially with decreasing ambient pressure. Such an extrapolation turns the curves in Figure 1a down through the origin at zero ambient pressure. Intuitively, an exponential extrapolation of critical tensions through the origin is more conservative than the linear extrapolation, since corresponding critical tensions for given ambient pressure are smaller, also noted by Ingle. If the extrapolation of critical tensions is allowed to follow the same exponential decrease of ambient pressure with altitude, then the ratio of the critical tension over ambient pressure, R, remains constant. Non-stop time limits in the exponential scheme are also smaller than corresponding time limits in the linear scheme. As seen in Table 2, atmospheric pressure falls off approximately 3.5% for every 1000 *ft* of elevation. Exponential extrapolations of critical tensions were tested by Bassett, and recently discussed by Ingle, the basis for operational procedures suggested by Cross, Smith, and Wienke. Correlations of altitude chokes data for goats with constant ratio, R, trigger points have been described by Lanphier.

2.4 DIFFUSION MODEL

Some researchers feel that only one tissue type is responsible for marginal symptoms of decompression sickness, a suggestion actually dating back to the early times of Haldane. Adopting the approach of Hill, in which extravascular tissue is regarded as a flat parallel slab bathed on both sides by arterial blood, Hempleman suggested that a single tissue approach to decompression should prove satisfactory. Abandoning perfusion limited gas exchange also, diffusion in a fully-stirred medium was assumed instead. Popular belief that blood perfusion is the only dominant mechanism for controlling dissolved gas exchange in critical tissues was challenged by Hills and Hempleman, following analyses of nitrogen and helium bends thresholds for bounce diving. At this point, it is fair to say that both play a role in critical tissues, and that both have been used in fabricating decompression tables, with a diffusion model the basis of the Royal Navy tables. Additionally, bulk diffusion models suggest a depth-time law restricting bounce exposures, notably lending some credence to their validity.

Like perfusion, diffusion limited gas exchange is also modeled in time by exponential response functions, bounded by arterial and initial tissue tensions, described in Appendix B. However, instead of many tissue compartments, a single bulk tissue is assumed in calculations, characterized by a gas diffusion constant, *D*. Tissue is separated into intravascular (blood) and extravascular (cells) regions. Blood containing dissolved inert and metabolic gases passes through the intravascular zone, providing initial and boundary conditions for subsequent gas diffusion into the extravascular zone. A diffusion equation describes the spatial and temporal behavior of the inert gas as it migrates between blood and tissue. Solutions are expanded as a Fourier series in space and time and resulting terms are averaged in space over the tissue regions for a bulk response. The overall response looks like an averaged sum of multi-tissue components, varying as $\tau/(2n - 1)^2$ and weighted by the same factor, $1/(2n - 1)^2$, for n a positive integer.

A critical phase gradient, *G*, is used to limit exposures, with *G* the difference between nitrogen tension (absolute units) and ambient pressure, *P*. Rashbass suggested a fixed $G = 30$ *fsw*, but such a critical gradient is too conservative for deep and bounce exposures and not conservative enough for shallow and saturation exposures. Later, Hempleman introduced a depth dependent critical gradient, *G*, supplanting the fixed gradient, providing the means to parameterize bounce and saturation diving in the same model framework, seen in Figure 2. Such bulk diffusion models are attractive theoretically because they permit the whole diving profile to be modeled with one equation. And a very important feature of bulk diffusion treatments is the $t^{1/2}$ behavior of gas uptake and elimination in time, *t*. Linked to data, diffusion models require a $t^{1/2}$ variation of bounce time limits with depth.

As shown in Appendix B, diffusion models limit gas uptake and elimination by a number of factors, such as the tissue thickness, *l*, diffusivity, *D*, depth of exposure, *d*, initial tissue tension, and time. For relatively short times, Hempleman limited non-stop time limits, t_s, according to the depth, *d*, by requiring $dt_s^{1/2} \leq 475$ *fsw* min$^{1/2}$. Such a law follows directly from the structure of the bulk diffusion equation, and challenges the previous perfusion dominated formulation. In fairness to both schemes, a way around the controversy was suggested by Hills and Hennessy in formulating the blood flow and gas exchange mechanism as a two step perfusion plus diffusion process. Discussion of that model will follow. For perspective, it is noted that the non-stop US Navy limits satisfy a modified relationship, that is, $dt_s^{1/2} \leq 500$ *fsw* min$^{1/2}$. Similarly, based on reductions in counts of venous gas emboli, Spencer later suggested that the constant be reduced, that is, $dt_s^{1/2} \leq 465$ *fsw* min$^{1/2}$.

Such predictive success in parameterizing bounce diving is quite noteworthy. As a dissolved gas model, many believe that much of its success hinges on the relative absence of appreciable free phases during

Figure 2. Diffusion Limited Critical Gradient.

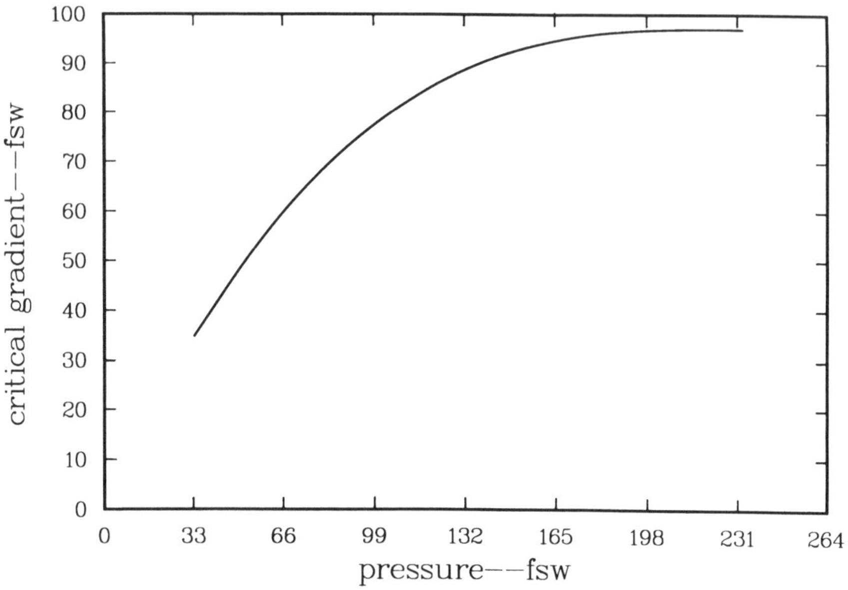

A single tissue is assumed in diffusion models, characterized by a diffusion coefficient, D. The difference between the tissue tension and ambient pressure is limited by the critical gradient, G, depicted above. In terms of a critical tension, M, we have $G = M/.79 - P$ in absolute units. Diffusion models exhibit a characteristic $t^{1/2}$ temporal behavior for gas uptake and elimination, serving as the basis for the Hempleman exposure law,

$$dt_s^{1/2} \leq 475 \text{ fsw min}^{1/2},$$

with t_s the non-stop time limit, and d the depth.

bounce exposures. When applied to multi-diving, the diffusion model experiences difficulties not unlike those described for perfusion models, probably for the same basic reasons, namely free phases. Because diffusion models are also single tissue, they do not possess the same flexibility as multi-tissue models insofar as data fitting. For some, this is a shortcoming, for others, a firmer theoretical basis.

2.5 VARIANTS AND HYBRIDS

Extensions of basic (perfusion and diffusion) models redress some of the deficiencies, both in theory and application. Concerns about microbubbles in the blood impacting gas elimination, geometry of the tissue region with respect to gas exchange, penetration depths for gas diffusion, nerve deformation trigger points for pain, gas uptake and elimination asymmetry, effective gas exchange with flowing blood, and perfusion-versus-diffusion limited gas exchange, to name but a few, motivated a number of modifications.

The multi-tissue model addresses dissolved gas transport with saturation gradients driving the elimination. In the presence of free phases, free-dissolved and free-blood elimination gradients can compete with dissolved-blood gradients. Wienke suggested that the gradient be split into two weighted parts, the free-blood and dissolved-blood gradients, with the weighting fraction proportional to the amount of separated gas per unit tissue volume. Use of a split gradient is consistent with multi-phase flow partitioning, and implies that only a portion of tissue gas has separated, with the remainder dissolved. Such a split representation could replace any of the gradient terms in tissue response functions in any model.

If gas nuclei are entrained in the circulatory system, blood perfusion rates are effectively lowered, and impairment with impact on all gas exchange processes. Albano and others suggested lengthening the tissue half-lives for elimination over those for uptake, for instance a 10 *minute* compartment for uptake becomes a 12 *minute* compartment on elimination. Such lengthening procedure and the split elimination gradient obviously render gas uptake and elimination processes as asymmetric. In a similar vein, Thalmann and Spaur suggested another asymmetical scheme. Instead of both exponential uptake and elimination, exponential uptake and linear elimination response functions are chosen. Such modifications can be employed in any perfusion model quite easily, and tuned to the data.

In simple diffusion models, planar (slab) geometry is assigned to the blood-tissue interface and extended region. Considering the radial symmetry of blood flow through vessels in tissue, cylindrical (Krogh) geometry is more appropriate. Roughton and Wittenborn, among others, extended the slab model to one-dimensional cylindrical geometry (Appendix B), with spatial average over cylindrical annuli yielding Bessel function weighting factors. The geometrical effects of planar versus cylindrical geometry are in the 6-12% range for bulk models, that is, impacting gas uptake and elimination. In the cylindrical case, time constants in the exponentials link to the dimensions of the tissue zone.

Hempleman assumed a uniform tissue region characterized by a single diffusion coefficient, D. Both fixed and depth dependent critical gradients were employed in analyses. Nishi introduced a variant of that model by breaking the extended tissue zone into four serial compartments with the same bulk diffusivity, but different critical ratios, R, or tensions, M. Critical parameters are fixed across all depths, and are correlated with venous gas emboli measurements. This model forms the basis of the DCIEM (Canadian) tables. Gas will sequentially penetrate each compartment according to the appropriate diffusion time across preceding compartments.

Questions of whether perfusion or diffusion are actually rate limiting in critical tissues, whether bounded (finite spatial dimension) or bulk (infinite or averaged-over spatial dimension) are sufficiently representative for decompression analysis, how are dissolved-free gas interactions best quantified for table and meter algorithms, and why are seemingly dissimilar models almost equally successful in applications, prompted studies with broader kinetic perspectives. By the 1970s, accessiblity to high speed computers permitted the numerical resolution of extremely complex problems, augmenting analyses on the computational side. Perfusion-diffusion models are an offspring of such studies and activities, and the modeling work of Hills and Hennessy is notable, coupling blood flow and tissue gas diffusion in a complicated, but comprehensive, framework. For many, the perfusion-diffusion exchange model is the standard, recovering the rate limiting features of perfusion or diffusion in appropriate circumstance.

The *thermodynamic* approach suggested by Hills, and extended by Hennessy, is more comprehensive than any earlier models, addressing a number of issues simultaneously, such as tissue gas exchange, phase separation, and phase volume trigger points. This model is based on phase equilibration of dissolved and separated gas phases, with temporal uptake and elimination of inert gas controlled by perfusion and diffusion. From a boundary (vascular) zone of thickness, *a*, gases diffuse into the cellular region. Radial, one-dimensional, cylindrical geometry is assumed for simplicity, as described in Appendix B. Diffusion is controlled by the difference between the instantaneous tissue tension and the venous tension, and perfusion is controlled by the difference between the arterial and venous tension. A mass balance for gas flow at the vascular-cellular interface, *a*, enforces the perfusion limit when appropriate, linking the diffusion and perfusion equations directly. Blood and tissue tensions are joined in a complex feedback loop. The trigger point in the thermodynamic model is the separated phase volume, related to a set of mechanical pain thresholds for fluid injected into connective tissue. Details are presented in Appendix C.

In parallel analysis, considering both radial and axial gas transport, Hennessy showed that the solution to the coupled perfusion-diffusion set of equations in various limits recovered the solutions to all deterministic models hitherto proposed and studied for gas exchange.

The full thermodynamic model is complex, but yet Hills has performed massive computations and correlations with data, underscoring its operational validity. One of its more significant features can be seen in Figure 4. Considerations of free phase dynamics (phase volume trigger point) require deeper decompression staging formats, compared to considerations of critical tensions, and are characteristic of phase models. Full blown bubble models require the same, simply to minimize bubble excitation and growth. These models follow, but before considering them, application of the popular Haldane model is detailed across a spectrum of activity.

CHAPTER 3

Typical Applications

In applying models and equations, we are faced with either fitting data to situations using plausible bases, or synthesizing mathematical models based strategically on first principles. Present practice relies on the former, and calculational methods target a limited range of conditions. With that understanding, we can launch into specific application of the Haldane model. In presenting gas buildup and elimination curves, square wave profiles, assuming maximum gas tension over any time interval of interest, will be employed for graphical simplicity, and without loss of generality.

In compressed air diving, nitrogen tensions are measured in weight fractions of ambient (absolute) pressure, with nitrogen fraction the usual 0.79. By conventions, both pressures and depths are measured in feet-of-sea-water *(fsw)*. Degrees to which compartments tolerate supersaturation are limited by critical values, *M*, fitted to the historical data by straight lines, depicted in Figure 1a, with τ, M_0, and ΔM tabulated in Table 1. They are representative of multi-tissue sets employed in tables and meters. Ranges of variation are neither large, nor diverse in application. How they are employed, that is, their implementation across a spectrum of exposures, also does not vary theoretically from table to meter. Self-consistency is somewhat a keynote, though claims about advantages of particular sets of tissue parameters can be made on bases of test ranges, statistics, and correlations.

Parameter sets and critical values derive from data fits, iterative repetitions, hindsight, possibly venous gas emboli correlations, and bootstrapping of earlier models. Ranges are bounded, as are permissible activities. If extended to altitude, the surfacing limits M_0, decrease either exponentially (very rapidly) or linearily (more gradually). With notable parameter leeway in Table 1, additional leeway in permissible ascent and descent rates, and a set of non-stop time limits, a multiplicity of (safe) schedules are possible within the model framework. After testing, such schedules would then be fit for general diving consumption. Similar comments apply to the software driving any digital meter, effectively employing some equivalent version of Table 1.

Repetitive and decompression diving must contend with a greater fraction of separated gas. And this makes extrapolations of bounce diving fits more difficult. In the early days, slower tissue compartments were added to accommodate deeper, prolonged, and decompression exposures. Ostensibly, slower compartments might track a greater proportion of separated gas, possibly dumped from tissues into gas micronuclei. Laboratory studies in decompressed gels bear witness to typical growth and elimination patterns in gas nuclei and bubbles spanning hours. Of course, bubbles and nuclei in the body are both perfused and metabolic, adding to complexity. While not always optimal, tissue response functions with very slow compartments can be coupled to critical tensions for repetitive diving. The approach is more limited for repetitive diving than bounce diving, as possibly witnessed by higher bends incidence in divers embarking on multi-day and repetitive activity, according to Vann and Dovenbarger. In such repetitive application, tables and meters which do not accommodate slower compartments, like $\tau > 60$ minutes, appear further limited. For that very reason, the US Navy expanded the original set some fifty years ago, replacing the 70 minute compartment with an 80 minute compartment and adding the 120 minute compartment. Yet, the tendency today to add compartments in the several hundred minutes range, while well-intentioned, is probably not the best means for tracking separated phases. Very slow compartments, in the several hundred minute range, cannot really control multi-day and heavy repetitive diving by tracking just dissolved phases. Present consensus thus cautions against 3 or more repetitive dives in any 24 hour period, especially in the deeper categories (beyond 100 *fsw*), and relaxation periods of at least a day following 3-4 days of repetitive activity.

3.1 BOUNCE DIVING

In bounce diving, exposures at depth for any time are followed by immediate return to the surface. Accordingly, consider a bounce dive to 60 *fsw* for 40 *minutes,* an exposure in the no-stop category for tables and meters. Figure 3a depicts both gas uptake (solid line) in the 20 minute compartment as a function of time and corresponding *M* (dotted line) throughout the exposure, neglecting the time to surface from 60 *fsw*, and thus any outgassing during the interval. Note that at no time underwater nor at the surface, is *M* exceeded by the tissue tension, the case in all compartments for this exposure. Bounce diving within dissolved gas models is well parameterized.

Figure 3a. Tissue And Critical Tensions (60 fsw/40 minutes).

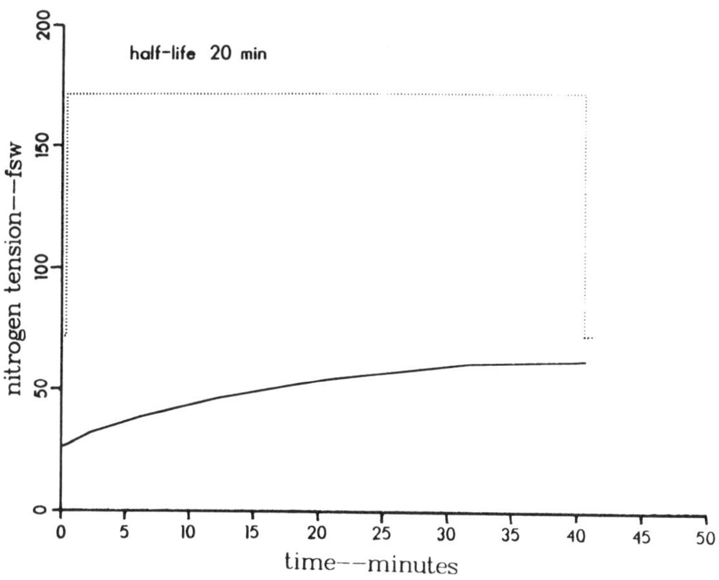

A dive to 60 fsw for 40 minutes is a no-stop dive. Here the critical tensions for the 20 minute compartment (dotted line) are plotted against the tissue tensions (solid line). Critical tensions are never exceeded. Such is also the case in all other compartments.

But, suppose we lengthen the exposure to 70 *minutes,* certainly a decompression dive. Figure 3b contrasts nitrogen uptake against M for the 40 minute compartment, should the diver surface immediately after 70 *minutes*. While M is not exceeded at 60 *fsw*, the surfacing limit M_0 is exceeded. Clearly this diver would need to first decompress before surfacing. Here, only the 40 minute compartment is impacted. In general more than one compartment can be affected by exposures exceeding the no-stop time limits. If the diver, after 70 *minutes* at 60 *fsw,* makes a stop at 10 *fsw* for 2 *minutes,* he could safely ascend to the surface. The profile for the 40 minute compartment is depicted in Figure 3c in that case. Again, critical tensions are not exceeded.

3.2 REPETITIVE DIVING

The Haldane approach to repetitive diving parallels that for bounce diving. Critical tensions again limit permissible degrees of compartment saturation. As an example of both repetitive application and diving idiom, *deepest*

Figure 3b. Tissue And Critical Tensions (60 fsw/70 minutes).

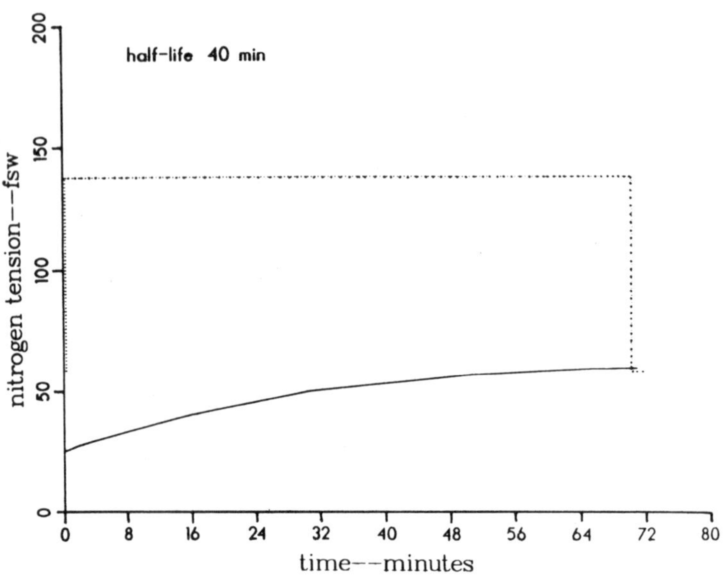

A dive to 60 fsw for 70 minutes is a decompression exposure. In this case, the surfacing critical tension, M_0, is exceeded in the 40 minute compartment. In decompression exposures, more than one compartment may be affected.

dive first, consider the profiles in Figures 3d and 3e for the 40 minute compartment. In the first case (Figure 3d), an exposure to 70 *fsw* for 45 minutes is followed by a surface interval of 35 minutes, and then another dive to 50 *fsw* for 35 minutes. In the second case (Figure 3e), the order is reversed, that is 50 *fsw* for 35 minutes, 35 minutes of surface interval, followed by 70 *fsw* for 45 minutes. Clearly, the first repetitive case is a no-stop exposure, while the second is not. In Figure 3d, critical tensions are not exceeded, while in Figure 3e, the critical tension, M_0, is compromised at the end of the dive.

Repetitive application of dissolved gas models does not enjoy the same success as bounce diving application. Free phases in tissues have had some time to grow between dives, and the next dive then pumps in a fresh supply of dissolved gas, possibly feeding phase growth if elimination has not been effective.

3.3 MULTI-LEVEL DIVING

Multi-level diving presents additional challenges to the classical scheme, though most problems occur with table usage, and less so with

Figure 3c. Tissue And Critical Tensions (60 fsw/70 minutes, 10 fsw/2 minutes).

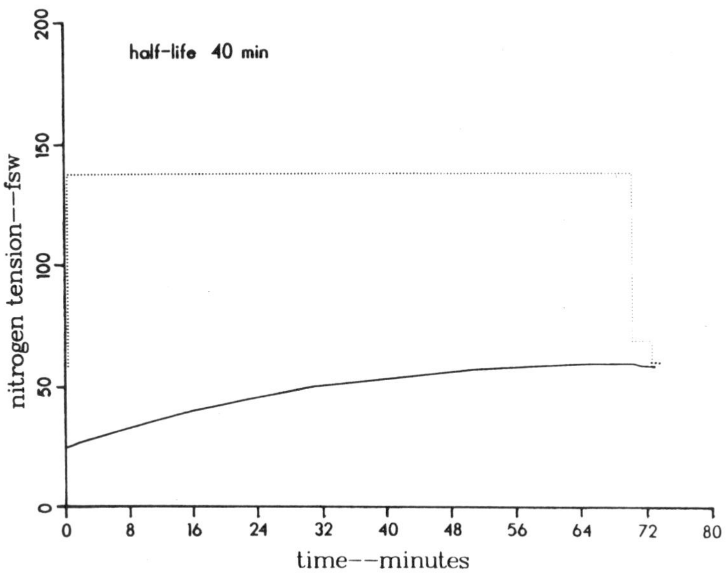

If the exposure at 60 fsw for 70 minutes is followed by a decompression stop at 10 fsw for 2 minutes, tissue tensions in the 40 minute compartment are maintained below critical tensions at all times. Other compartment tensions are also maintained below critical tensions.

digital devices. The reason is not too complicated. Tables generally rely on the slowest tissue compartment to dictate staging and repetitive formats. Repetitive intervals are chosen so that the faster compartments cannot control the exposure upon surfacing, with 10 minutes the usual limit. Tables cannot account for gas uptake or elimination in faster compartments for shorter time intervals, and thus request that shorter time intervals be added directly to exposure times. In multi-level table application, the 10 minute interval is neglected, and gas exchange in the faster compartments is not considered. At times, neglect of the faster compartments causes trouble, especially when their critical tensions are exceeded with the tables blind for some 10 minutes. Because meters continuously monitor activities in all compartments, these table concerns are minimized in multi-level excursions. While such a problem is more an implementation issue than fundamental issue, foregoing concerns in bounce, repetitive, and decompression exposures still carry over here.

As a comparison of multi-level table and meter diving, consider Figure 3f. Tissue and critical tensions in the 10 minute compartment for a multi-level

Figure 3d. Tissue And Critical Tensions (70 fsw/45 minutes, surface/ 35 minutes, 50 fsw/35 minutes).

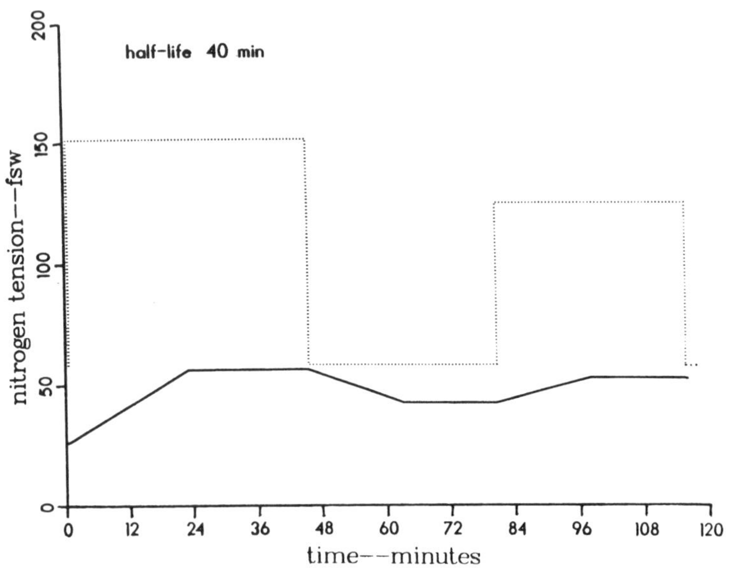

If the deepest segment (70 fsw/45 minutes) of the repetitive exposure is performed first, followed by a surface interval and the shallow segment (50 fsw/35 minutes) critical tensions are not exceeded in the compartments, as seen for the 40 minute tissue.

exposure are depicted. The exposure consists of three segments, 120 *fsw* for 12 minutes, 90 *fsw* for 10 minutes, and 80 *fsw* for 2 minutes. According to the USN tables, the profile is marginally safe. But, according to Figure 3f, the surfacing critical tension, M_0, is violated. A meter could arrest this problem before it occurred, while a table might exhibit marginal indifference (depending on user discretion).

Systematically deeper-to-shallow diving practices are optimal in all cases. Deeper-than-previous excursions have the potential to excite smaller, more stable, gas nuclei into growth. Deeper-spike and sawtooth diving profiles become more hazardous as repetitive frequency increases, likely due to the presence of growing bubbles and excitable gas nuclei in slower tissues and slingshot effect of higher tensions surrounding them.

Though not formally validated, schemes for multi-level diving, particularly within the US Navy tables, have been proposed. Some are employed in the commercial, scientific, and sport sectors. One popular approach employs back-to-back repetitive sequencing, assigning groups at the start of each multi-level dive, based on the total bottom time (actual plus residual nitrogen) of the previous segment. At times, that method allows critical tensions, other than the controlling 120 minute compartment tension, to be exceeded upon surfacing. But by tightening the exposure window, such a multi-level technique can be made consistent with the permissible tension formulation of the US Navy tables. In studying this multi-level technique, Wienke and Graver drew a line (envelope) across the US Navy tables, separating dives violating at least one critical tension at some point in the multi-level sequence from those not violating any critical tensions. Ascent and descent rates of 60 *ft/min* were also included in calculations. Some 16 million multi-level dives were analyzed on a CRAY supercomputer, employing the US Navy (Workman) set of tissue half-lives and critical tensions.

The envelope moves non-stop time limits back a group or more in the US Navy tables, restricting the back-to-back repetitive method in the same measure. Resulting multi-level restrictions are straightforward, simple for possible testing. Within a 130 *fsw* depth constraint, zonal limits and exposure restrictions in extreme cases are listed, depending on initial depth in the sequence:

(1) 100 - 130 *fsw* for 8 *minutes,* 80 - 100 *fsw* for 12 *minutes,* 60 - 80 *fsw* for 5 *minutes,* 50 - 60 *fsw* for 5 *minutes,* 40 - 50 *fsw* for 10 *minutes,* and 0 - 40 *fsw* for 20 *minutes;*

(2) 80 - 100 *fsw* for 22 *minutes,* 60 - 80 *fsw* for 5 *minutes,* 50 - 60 *fsw* for 5 *minutes,* 40 - 50 *fsw* for 10 *minutes,* and 0 - 40 *fsw* for 20 *minutes;*

(3) 60 - 80 *fsw* for 35 *minutes,* 50 - 60 *fsw* for 5 *minutes,* 40 - 50 *fsw* for 10 *minutes,* and 0 - 40 *fsw* for 20 *minutes;*

(4) 50 - 60 *fsw* for 55 *minutes,* 40 - 50 *fsw* for 10 *minutes,* and 0 - 40 *fsw* for 20 *minutes;* and,

(5) 40 - 50 *fsw* for 80 *minutes,* and 0 - 40 *fsw* for 20 *minutes.*

Within these times, the diver may theoretically ascend directly to the surface, since tissue tensions in all compartments are below critical tensions. Such zonal limits roughly correspond to the depth ranges of various controlling tissue compartments (5, 10, 20, 40, 80, and 120 *minutes).*

3.4 SATURATION DIVING

Like bounce diving, saturation diving, especially with mixed gases, has received considerable attention. Following exposures near 12 *hrs,* all

Figure 3e. Tissue And Critical Tensions (50 fsw/35 minutes, surface/ 35 minutes, 70 fsw/45 minutes).

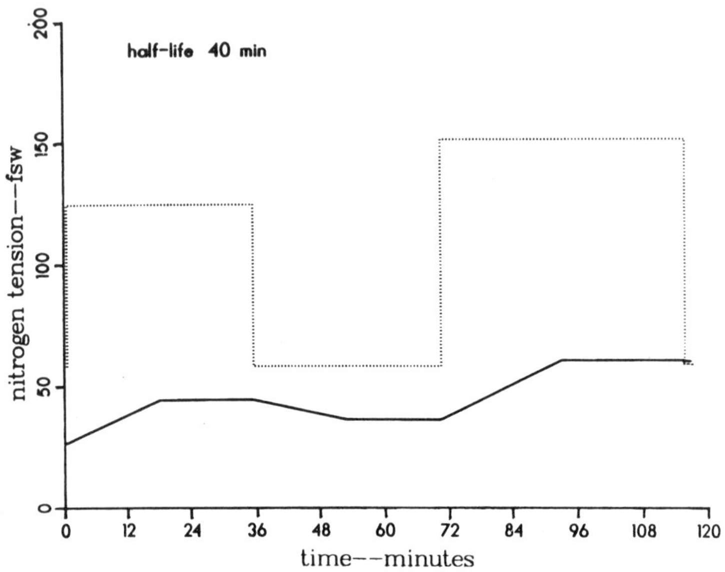

However, if the order of the repetitive segments in Figure 3d is reversed, the critical surfacing tension, M_0, is exceeded on ascent. Such is one reason for the well-known idiom "deepest dive first." In bubble theories, the practice will reduce possible excitation of smaller gas nuclei into growth.

compartments are essentially equilibrated with ambient pressure. Ascent is then controlled by the slowest compartment, the one with the smallest critical tension, *M*. Compartments with half-lives in the range, $120 \leq \tau \leq 720$ *minutes*, are usually employed. In spite of compartment structure chosen, an interesting feature, consistent with Figure 5, arises in terms of critical tension in the slowest compartments.

From experiments, the saturation curve, relating permissible tissue tension to ambient pressure, has been well established for almost any gas mixture. In the case of air, Figure 5 depicts that relationship in absolute units, that is, $Q = M/.79$ versus *P*. In terms of a linear *M* the saturation air curve requires $M_0 \approx 44$ *fsw*, while $\Delta M \approx 1.06$. While time scales for ascent vary according to the half-life of the slowest compartment, critical tensions for saturation staging vary slightly. Similar structure is seen in diffusion algorithms, employing a critical gradient, *G*. For example, in the Royal Navy tables, Rashbass first employed a fixed gradient, $G = 30$ *fsw,* compared to $(M_0/.79 - 33) = 23$ *fsw* in Figure 5. Later, Hempleman reduced the surfacing gradient, $G = 20$ *fsw*. As seen in Appendix B, the equivalent tissue half-life

Figure 3f. Tissue And Critical Tensions (120 fsw/12 minutes,90 fsw/10 minutes, 80 fsw/2 minutes).

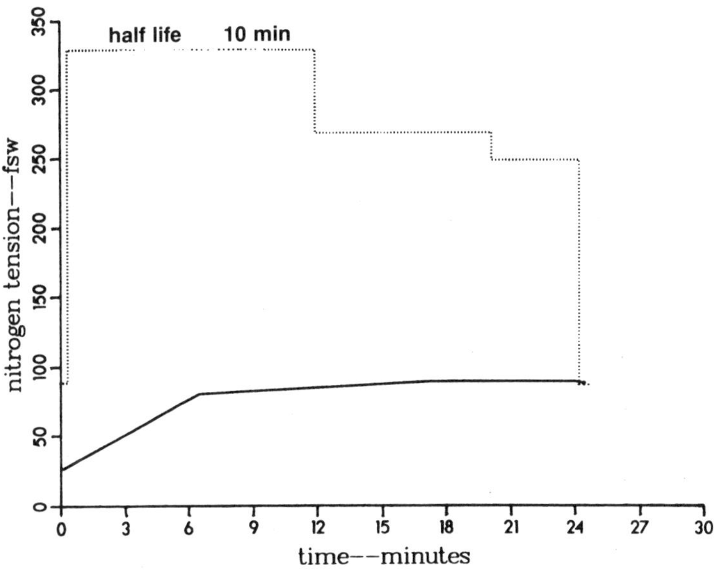

A table-safe (marginally) multi-level dive is shown to be unsafe according to instantaneous meter calculations. Tables are sometimes blind for short intervals of time (minimum repetitive interval) when tissue tensions in fast compartments may exceed critical values, as seen in the 10 minute compartment.

for the diffusion algorithm is 87 *minutes.* In short, no matter what the table or model, saturation staging formats are usually consistent with the saturation curve shown in Figure 5, more particularly, the slope and intercept. In that sense, all models collapse to a slow, single tissue equivalent, as discussed by Hennessy and Hempleman. For bounce diving, of course, models vary in their tissue number, critical parameters, or trigger points.

3.5 ALTITUDE DIVING

Tables and meters designed for sea level need be conservatively modified at altitude if possible, otherwise, not employed. Decomputer and table use are best left to manufacturer and designer discretions, but in any case, modification of critical tensions is central to any Haldane altitude algorithm. We will describe a general technique and, for discussion purposes, the USN dive tables (or derivative) will suffice.

Present diving schedules are based to large extent on the model discussed in the previous section, constraining activities so that *M* or *R* are never compromised. An approach to altitude diving that is roughly as conservative as the tested schemes of Buhlmann, and Bell and Borgwardt, holds the ratios, *R,* constant at altitude, forcing altitude exposures to be *similar* to sea level exposures, as seen in Appendix A. Such similarity will force *M* to decrease exponentially with increasing altitude, keeping *R* constant with commensurate exponential reduction in the ambient pressure, *P.* Constant *R* extrapolations of this sort should be confined to light diving activities, certainly not heavy repetitive, decompression, nor saturation exposures where they are not applicable.

The sought ratio constancy, *R*, at altitude induces a necessary scaling of actual depths to sea level equivalent depths for table entry, while all times remain unchanged. Actual depths at altitude are multiplied by factors, α, called altitude correction factors, which are just the ratios of sea level ambient pressure to altitude ambient pressure. Today, accurate wrist altimeters facilitate rapid, precise estimation of α on site. They are simply estimated from the *barometer* equation and are always greater than one. Table 2 lists correction factors in multiples of 1000 *fsw.* The higher one ascends to dive, the deeper is his relative exposure in terms of sea level equivalent depth. As with ambient pressure, relative increases of correction factors hasten rapidly above 10000 *ft.* From Table 2, *P* and α are seen to be reciprocally related, inverses actually. Again, time is measured directly, that is, correction factors are only applied to underwater depths, ascent rates, and stops. Equivalent approaches have been discussed in the past by Cross, Smith, and Bassett. Connection between constant *R* and exponentially decreasing *M* was later delineated by Wienke.

The similarity rule for altitude table modification and applying correction factors to calculations is straightforward. Convert depths at altitude to sea

Table 2. Altitude Correction Factors And USN Altitude Groups.

altitude, or change *(ft)*	ambient pressure *P (fsw)*	correction factor α	penalty group on arrival at altitude	permissible group for ascension to altitude
0	33.00	1.000		
1000	31.86	1.036	A	L
2000	30.77	1.072	B	K
3000	29.67	1.112	B	J
4000	28.55	1.156	C	I
5000	27.50	1.200	D	H
6000	26.53	1.244	E	G
7000	25.45	1.292	E	F
8000	24.55	1.344	F	E
9000	23.63	1.396	G	D
10000	22.72	1.452	H	C

level equivalent depths through multiplication by α. Convert all table sea level stops and ascent rates back to actual altitude through division by α. Ascent rates are always less than 60 *fsw/min,* while stops are always less than at sea level. Thus, a diver at 60 *fsw* at an elevation of 5000 *fsw* uses a depth correction of 72 *fsw,* taking $\alpha = 1.2$. Corresponding ascent rate is 50 *fsw/min,* and a stop at 10 *fsw* at sea level translates to 8 *fsw.*

If a diver has equilibrated with ambient pressure at any elevation, then any reduction in ambient pressure will put the diver in a repetitive group, merely because tissue tensions exceed ambient pressure. If the original and new pressures are specified, it is possible to estimate tissue saturation and, hence, repetitive group for the excursion. Similar comments apply to pressure reductions following any diving activity, with sea level diving the usual bill of fare. These considerations are treated as follows.

At sea level, each repetitive group represents an increment of tissue pressure over ambient ($P = 33$ *fsw*). For the USN tables, this increment is 2 *fsw* (absolute). If we compute the difference between sea level pressure and altitude ambient pressure, and then scale the difference by the ratio of sea level ambient pressure to altitude ambient pressure (correction factor α), we can estimate the repetitive group in which a sea level diver finds himself following immediate ascent to altitude. These group specifications are listed in column 4 of Table 2, and represent penalty time for the excursion to altitude. Entries were computed using sea level as the baseline, but are also appropriate (conservative) for any excursion between differing elevations.

In similar fashion, excursions to higher altitude following diving are limited by tissue critical tensions, and minimal repetitive group designators can be attached to any planned excursion. For the 120 minute compartment, the surfacing critical tension (sea level) is 51 *fsw* (nitrogen pressure) from Table 1. To be safer, we take 47 *fsw* as the limiting tension, convert it to an absolute tension of 60 *fsw* (47/.79), and then inversely scale it to altitude by the ratio of sea level pressure to altitude pressure, that is, α. The resulting limiting tensions at altitude can then be converted to standard USN groups which are tabulated in column 5 of Table 2. Entries represent maximum permissible groups for immediate altitude excursions, and do not account for any travel time. Thus a diver would have to wait some length of time after a dive, until he dropped into the permissible group category, before ascending. The D $-$ *group* rule for flying after diving is seen as a subcase for an altitude excursion to 9000 *fsw* (maxium cabin pressure).

Such is the regimen underlying dissolved gas decompression calculations for both tables and digital meters. Exposure possibilities are virtually infinite, spanning bounce to saturation, sea level to altitude, warm to cold water, sport to commercial, single to repetitive, and relaxed to strenuous diving. Over such range, and even before trying to factor diver and environmental factors into calculations, tables and meters are faced with a formidable task.

CHAPTER 4

Tables And Meters

Tables attempt to collate a broad category of exposures, such as the previous, with a minimal set of restricting, but safe, prescriptions. Calculations must encompass a maximum set of exposures for an optimal format. In addressing generality, achieving optimality is difficult. Groups of exposures within certain depth and time limits can be targeted by calculations for increments of 10 *fsw* and 10 *minutes*, the bases of many tables. Smaller increments would certainly provide greater reliability, but at the expense of brevity. And here is where meters can then shine. With the ability to instantaneously calculate tensions, meters continuously monitor diving activity in ways that tables cannot approach. Furthermore, for instantaneous values of tissue and critical tensions across all compartments, meters can then turn around and *invert* equations to estimate minimal time for safe ascension to shallower depth, albeit direct or staged ascent. When a compartment tension exceeds criticality, the meter is programmed to signal the diver to descend until the instantaneous tension falls beneath the critical tension, *M*.

Table and computer algorithms are only as realistic as the biophysical model upon which they are based. And that model is elusive, the object of scrutiny in recent years. From an operational viewpoint, the algorithm originally proposed by Haldane forms the basis for many dive tables and meters. Based on empirical limits for dissolved gases across phenomenological tissue compartments, which can be backfitted to almost any set of exposure data, the model is flexible, but skirts some issues contributing to limitations. So long as the range of exposure data to which the algorithm is tested and fitted is not exceeded in application, table and meter implementations are broadly equivalent. Meters do have the potential to optimize implementations since they function in continuous time modes, instantaneously folding information into calculations in ways that traditional tables cannot hope to emulate. In that sense, meters can be one up on tables. On the down side, some divers on computers are pushing the algorithm to the limits, with increases in bends incidence, particularly in the multi-day, multi-level, and repetitive categories where the algorithm has not been completely tested. If pushed to the very same limits, table usage would probably incur similar statistics. The problem is not one of tables versus meters, but rather algorithm versus testing.

4.1 VALIDATION

Testing is central to diving, and much testing of bounce (single), non-stop diving has transpired. Repetitive and multi-day exposures can neither claim, nor reap, the same benefits, and application of the algorithm in the latter cases has witnessed higher bends statistics than in the former one. Reasons, impacting modeling, can be conjectured. Most tables and meters use dissolved gas models, and so long as the bulk of tissue gas remains in the dissolved state, the more correct and useful will prove such approaches. But as increasing proportion of free phases grow, by direct excitation of critical micronuclei or more gradual bubble coalescing transitions, the algorithm can lose predictive capability. Invariably, such conditions attend diving activity *extrapolated* outside model and test ranges, sometimes as a surprise.

Certainly any algorithm can be piecewise safe over tested ranges, but not always globally. Some implementations, as pointed out by Weathersby and Homer, may not be statistically rigorous, relying on much too small a set of exposure data to confidently predict outcome. Models not strongly correlated with tests can promulgate wide variation in predictive capability. Similarly, models can often *interpolate* within data, while failing to *extrapolate* outside the data. And then we must modify procedures to accommodate the extrapolation. A good point in question is the repetitive use of the USN tables. It is now clear that single, no-stop (bounce) dives, followed possibly by one more repetitive dive, form the test basis of the non-stop parts of the schedules. Yet, we observe that multiple repetitive dives permitted by the tables incur higher bends statistics, particularly in the deeper categories. This results from both model shortcomings and less reliable statistics. Adequate testing of any algorithm is always requisite, that is, descent rate, exposure profile, ascent rate, surface interval, and repetitive loading, as reiterated by Schreiner and Hamilton. And, because differences in diver response have been noted in hyperbaric chambers and open water, for the same schedules, questions of wet versus dry testing are valid. As discussed in the last section, statistically significant testing, at the few percent level of incidence, usually requires some 20-40 trials.

4.2 OPERATIONAL PROCEDURES

Operational diving often requires many dives to various depths over periods of hours, and often days. Once a standard set of decompression tables has been constructed, with bounce diving the special case of non-stop decompression, a repetitive dive procedure is a necessity. After any air dive, variable amounts of residual nitrogen remain in body tissues for periods of 24 *hours* and more. Similarly, elevated tissue tensions can promote, or sustain, bubble growth over the same time scales. This residual gas (dissolved and free) buildup will shorten the exposure time for subsequent repetitive dives. The longer and deeper the first dive, the greater the amount of residual tissue nitrogen affecting decompression on subsequent dives. Non-stop depth-time allowances for repetitive dives are reduced in such circumstance. In bubble models, residual free gas phases are also included in procedures, imposing additional constraints on repetitive diving.

The many possibilities are easily tracked in continuous time mode by computers, as mentioned, but tables face a more difficult task. One approach, developed by Workman, groups combinations of depth and exposure times according to the surfacing tension in the slowest compartment. Then it is possible to account for desaturation during any arbitrary surface interval. The remaining excess nitrogen at the start of the next dive can always be converted into equivalent time spent at the deepest point of the dive. The so-called penalty time can then be added to actual dive time to compute appropriate tissue tensions.

Surfacing tensions in excess of 33 *fsw* (absolute) in the lowest compartment are assigned letter designations, A to O, for each 2 *fsw* over 33 *fsw*. Any, and all, exposures can be treated in this manner. To credit outgassing, a surface interval table, accounting for 2 *fsw* incremental drops in tensions in the slowest compartment, is also constructed. Such are the bases for the US Navy Air Decompression and Repetitive Surface Interval Tables, with the 120 *minute* compartment (the slowest) controlling repetitive activity. Standard USN tables provide safe procedures for dives up to 190 *fsw* for 60 *minutes*. Dives between 200 and 300 *fsw* were tested and reported in the exceptional exposure USN tables, including a 240 *minute* compartment. The Swiss tables, compiled by Buhlmann, incorporate the same basic procedures, but with a notable exception. While the US Navy tables were constructed for sea-level usage, requiring some safe extrapolation procedure to altitude as described, the Swiss tables are formulated and tested over a range of reduced ambient pressure. The controlling repetitive tissue in the Buhlmann, compilation is the 635 *minute* compartment.

Similar approaches focusing on deep and saturation diving have resulted in decompression tables for helium-oxygen, helium-oxygen-nitrogen, and even recent mixtures with some hydrogen. Inert gases other than nitrogen are employed to both reduce narcosis and speed elimination. Speedup roughly follows Graham's law, that is, elimination times scale inversely with the square root of the atomic weight, assuming simple molecular diffusion. That, of course, raises interesting questions regarding the dominance of perfusion or diffusion in controlling tissue gas exchange.

The Royal Navy took a different tack, employing a diffusion model. Following construction of an air decompression table, repetitive dives are referenced to the bottom time of the previous dive, the depth of the next dive, and the surface interval. Since only one tissue type is involved, it controls all exposures. Depth of a pair of dives is defined to be the deepest of the two, and any two dives performed within 2 *hrs* of each other use the combined bottom time of both. In repetitive application, the Hempleman-Rashbass approach is more conservative than the Workman or Buhlmann schemes.

While it is true that the table procedures just described are quite easily encoded in digital meters, and indeed such devices exist, digital meters are capable of much more than table recitations. Pulsing depth and pressure at short intervals, digital meters can monitor diving almost continuously, providing rapid estimates of any model parameter. When employing the exact same algorithms as tables, as seen in Figures 3a through 3f for the USN Haldane model, meters provide additional means to control and safety beyond usual table lookup. When model equations can be inverted in time, meters can easily compute time remaining before decompression, time at stop, surface interval before flying, and optimal ascent procedure. Profiles can be stored for later analysis, and the resulting data bank used to tune and improve models and procedures. Considering utility and functionality, meter usage should increase in diving, supported by technological advance in computing power, algorithmic sophistication, and general acceptance, though it will probably be some time though before tables are supplanted.

4.3 LIMITATIONS AND CAVEATS

We presently do not possess a first-principle decompression theory, but we suspect shortcomings of approaches and how to enhance their effective implementation. In the case of the dissolved gas algorithm, there are two problem areas, free phase dynamics and bends trigger points. Fundamentally, tissue tensions are not the same as gas pressures in bubbles and elimination gradients for dissolved phases are not the same as gradients for free phases. Alone, critical tensions cannot optimally address the most probable cause of bends (Type I and II), simply bubbles. With increased exposure, one deduces lower tolerance levels to free phases. With successively deeper profiles, one expects to excite greater numbers of gas nuclei into troublesome growth, exceeding body capacity for elimination. These considerations might root higher bends statistics, reported by the Divers Alert Network (DAN), for divers embarking on multi-day, repetitive, and multi-level excursions, in that order of decreasing risk. Bounce (non-repetitive) diving is relatively risk free these days, especially within algorithms employing reduced time limits which ostensibly restrict bubble growth. And the presence of only small proportions of free phases bootstraps dissolved gas model treatments, though such issues are best left to nucleation and bubble models. Safety stops and slower ascent rates also correlate in principle with bubble models as effective procedures. Further reduction in non-stop time limits appears a zero-sum game between safety and optimality.

Farm and Hayashi, Kunkle and Beckman, and Hills suggest that the empirical practices of Hawaiian and Australian diving fishermen (deeper decompression stops, zonal safety stops, and immediate in-water recompression) underscore working cognizance of phase dynamics developed over years of trial-and-error experimentation, albeit, with considerable trauma. Their practice seems to minimize phase growth apart from dissolved gas buildup. DAN reports that present diving practices appear riskier under increasing exposure time and pressure loading, spawning development of ancillary safety measures restricting multi-diving. Such measures are suggested within conservative table protocols, even for exposures not exceeding critical tensions. Accordingly, the following menu, used in conjunction with normal table and meter protocols, is prudent, and has been the subject of extensive discussion at recent workshops and technical forums sponsored by the American Academy of Underwater Sciences (AAUS) and the Undersea And Hyperbaric Medical Society (UHMS), as reported by Lang and Egstrom, Lang and Hamilton, and Sheffield:

(1) limit repetitive dives to a maximum of three per day, not exceeding the 100 *fsw* level;

(2) avoid multi-day, multi-level, or repetitive dives to increasing depths;

(3) wait 12 *hrs* before flying after nominal diving, 24 *hrs* after heavy diving (taxing, near decompression, or prolonged repetitive) activity, and 48 *hrs* after decompression diving;

(4) avoid multiple surface ascents and short repetitive dives *(spikes)* within surface intervals of 1 *hr;*

(5) surface intervals of more than an hour are recommended for repetitive diving;

(6) safety stops for 2-4 *minutes* in the 10-25 *fsw* zone are advisable for all diving, but particularly for deep (near 100 *fsw)*, repetitive, and multi-day exposures;

(7) do not dive at altitudes above 10000 *ft* using modified conventional tables, extrapolations, or constant decompression ratios.

Always dive conservatively, remembering that tables and meters are not *bends-proof.* Procedures such as those above are prudent, theoretically sound, and safe diving protocols. Ultimately, they can be linked to free phase and bubble concerns, addressed later within phase models. Before considering such models, it is worthwhile to examine some broad issues impacting decompression modeling.

CHAPTER 5

Issues

Mathematical models of inert gas transport and bubble formation all try to prevent decompression sickness. Developed over years of diving application, they differ on a number of basic issues, still mostly unresolved today:

(1) the rate limiting process for inert gas exchange (perfusion or diffusion);

(2) composition and location of critical tissues;

(3) the processes of phase inception and separation, leading to gas bubbles and decompression sickness;

(4) the critical trigger point (tension, separated phase volume, bubble number, inflation rate) best delimiting the onset of symptoms; and

(5) the nature of the critical insult (deformation, occlusion, ischemia, haemoconcentration).

Such issues confront every modeler and table designer, perplexing in their ambiguous correlations with experiment and nagging in their persistence. And here discussion is confined just to Type I and II bends, to say nothing of other types and factors. Some of these points have been mentioned, but a closer look is worthwhile.

5.1 PERFUSION AND DIFFUSION

Clearly in the foregoing, model distinctions were made on the basis of perfusion or diffusion limited gas exchange. The distinction is somewhat artificial, especially in light of the Hennessy and Hills analyses of coupled perfusion-diffusion gas transport. As mentioned, both studies recover limiting features of the exchange process in appropriate limits. The distinction is perhaps of passing interest today, but yet perfusion and diffusion limited algorithms are used in mutually exclusive fashion in diving. The obvious mathematical rigors of a full blown perfusion-diffusion treatment of gas exchange mitigate against table and meter implementation, where model simplicity is a necessity. So one or another limiting models is adopted, with inertia and track record sustaining use. Certainly Haldane models fall into that categorization. Still, within the context of just perfusion or diffusion limited gas exchange, a number of interesting anomalies arise, discussed by Kety and Schmidt, Hills, Tepper and Lightfoot, Jones, Thompson, Roughton, and Hempleman.

In multi-issue (Haldane) models, a nagging question of interpretation of a spectrum of critical tensions arises. If the hypothetical compartments represent local differences in circulation within the same anatomical tissue, they should have the same critical tension, as originally proposed by Haldane. But, if they represent different anatomical identities, then the same insult to different tissues should produce different clinical signs and manifestations, yet, the same set of symptoms occurs independent of the compartment affected. Some would argue that it is better to introduce critical tensions as variables depending on depth, time, temperature, and so on, while holding them independent of half-life. In single tissue models, of course, this happens *de facto*.

While the spectrum of half-lives in perfusion models is reasonable from the perspective of inert gas washout times, diffusion coefficients, *D*, assigned to model calculations, or extracted from data fits, are more ambiguous. In calculational models, gas diffusivities, *D*, in tissue are five orders of magnitude smaller than in water, comprising the bulk of tissue matter. Typical water diffusivities are on the order of 10^{-5} $cm^2\ sec^{-1}$, while model tissue values are near 10^{-10} $cm^2\ sec^{-1}$. In critical sites, anomalously reduced diffusion might be ascribed to geometry of the site, or composition of the tissue. Hills suggested cellular effects, while Hempleman was concerned about avascularity, both implying longer diffusion time scales.

Such questions, of course, suffer from the same problem common to other vital issues, namely identification of the critical tissue and site. Another way to look at the question of perfusion-versus-diffusion might be through the bounce data for different breathing mixtures. In bounce diving, selection of helium or nitrogen as the inert gas is a trade between the lower solubility, *S*, of helium, less than nitrogen by a factor of 3-5, and the greater diffusivity, *D*, about 2.7 times greater than nitrogen by Graham's law. For long exposure times, solubility factors dominate and helium is a better breathing gas than nitrogen. The solubility advantage should also hold up for short exposures if gas exchange is perfusion limited, while if diffusion is rate limiting, the 2.7 diffusion advantage of helium might be expected to outdistance its 3-5 solubility advantage over nitrogen, and so air (nitrogen) would be better for bounce diving. Goat experiments clearly show that nitrogen is better for bounce exposures of less than 20 *minutes* duration, that is, longer non-stop time limits compared to helium. The implication is then simple, namely that some gas uptake in critical tissues is diffusion limited.

But the controversy does not end there. An obvious way to differentiate between blood perfusion and diffusion is to measure the time it takes for inert gas to diffuse into tissue. Kety, Thompson, and Roughton measured this transit time, and found that the mean extravascular tension attained 95-99% of the blood tension in 1-5 *sec*. This is so very rapid that diffusion should not play a rate limiting role, that is, values of D smaller than water diffusivites are precluded.

5.2. BUBBLE SITES

We do not really know where bubbles form nor lodge, their migration patterns, their birth and dissolution mechanisms, nor the exact chain of physico-chemical insults resulting in decompression sickness. Many possibilities exist, differing in the nature of insult, the location, and the manifestation of symptoms. Bubbles might form directly *(de novo)* in supersaturated sites upon decompression, or possibly grow from preformed, existing seed nuclei excited by compression-decompression. Leaving their birth sites, bubbles may move to critical sites elsewhere. Or stuck at their birth sites, bubbles may grow locally to pain-provoking size. They might dissolve locally by gaseous diffusion to surrounding tissue or blood, or passing through screening filters, such as the lung complex, they might be broken down into smaller aggregates, or eliminated completely. Whatever the bubble history, it presently escapes complete elucidation.

Bubbles may hypothetically form in the blood (intravascular) or outside the blood (extravascular). Once formed, intravascularly or extravascularly, a number of critical insults are possible. Intravascular bubbles may stop in closed circulatory vessels and induce ischemia, blood sludging, chemistry degradations, or mechanical nerve deformation. Circulating gas emboli may occlude the arterial flow, clog the pulmonary filters, or leave the circulation to lodge in tissue sites as extravascular bubbles. Extravascular bubbles may remain locally in tissue sites, assimilating gas by diffusion from adjacent supersaturated tissue and growing until a nerve ending is deformed beyond its pain threshold. Or, extravascular bubbles might enter the arterial or venous flows, at which point they become intravascular bubbles.

Spontaneous bubble formation in fluids usually requires large decompressions, like hundreds of *atmospheres,* somewhere near fluid tensile limits. Many feel that such circumstance precludes direct bubble formation in blood following decompression. Explosive, or very rapid decompression, of course is a different case. But, while many doubt that bubbles form in the blood directly, intravascular bubbles have been seen in both the arterial and venous circulation, with vastly greater numbers detected in venous flows (venous gas emboli). Ischemia resulting from bubbles caught in the arterial network has long been implied as a cause of decompression sickness. Since the lungs are effective filters of venous bubbles, arterial bubbles would then most likely originate in the arteries or adjacent tissue beds. The more numerous venous bubbles, however, are suspected to first form in lipid tissues draining the veins. Lipid tissue sites also possess very few nerve endings, possibly masking critical insults. Veins, thinner than arteries, appear more susceptible to extravascular gas penetration.

Extravascular bubbles may form in aqueous (watery) or lipid (fatty) tissues in principle. For all but extreme or explosive decompression, bubbles are seldom observed in heart, liver, and skeletal muscle. Most gas is seen in fatty tissue, not unusual considering the five-fold higher solubility of nitrogen in lipid tissue versus aqueous tissue. Since fatty tissue has few nerve endings, tissue deformation by bubbles is unlikely to cause pain locally. On the other hand, formations or large volumes of extravascular gas could induce vascular hemorrhage, depositing both fat and bubbles into the circulation as noted in animal experiments. If mechanical pressure on nerves is a prime candidate for critical insult, then tissues with high concentrations of nerve endings are candidate structures, whether tendon or spinal cord. While such tissues are usually aqueous, they are invested with lipid cells whose propensity reflects total body fat. High nerve density and some lipid content supporting bubble formation and growth would appear a conducive environment for a mechanical insult.

On the question of preformed nuclei, their presence in human tissue has not been demonstrated. The existence of preformed nuclei in blood serum and egg albumin has been reported by Yount and Strauss. Since preformed nuclei are found virtually in every aqueous substance known, their preclusion from the body would come as a surprise to many. Hence, while most regard nucleation as a random process, its occurrence in tissue seems highly probable, seen for instance in the studies of Evans, Walder, Strauss, Yount, Kunkle, and co-workers. Model correlations with incidence statistics of decompression sickness in salmon, rats, and humans speak favorably for the nucleation concept.

5.3 COMPUTATIONAL ALGORITHMS AND COMPLEXITY

The establishment and evolution of gas phases, and possible bubble trouble, involves a number of distinct, yet overlapping, steps:

(1) nucleation and stabilization (free phase inception);

(2) supersaturation (dissolved gas buildup);

(3) excitation and growth (free-dissolved phase interaction);

(4) coalescense (bubble aggregation); and

(5) deformation and occlusion (tissue damage and ischemia).

Over the years, much attention has focused on supersaturation. Recent studies have shed much light on nucleation, excitation and bubble growth, even though *in vitro*. Bubble aggregation, tissue damage, ischemia, and the whole question of decompression sickness trigger points are difficult to quantify in any model, and remain obscure. Complete elucidation of the interplay is presently asking too much. Yet, the development and implementation of better computational models is necessary to address problems raised in workshops, reports, publications, disclaimers, and as a means to safer diving.

The computational issues of bubble dynamics (formation, growth, and elimination) are mostly outside the traditional framework, but get folded into half-life specifications in a non-tractable mode. The very slow tissue compartments (τ large, or D small) might be tracking both free and dissolved gas exchange in poorly perfused regions. Free and dissolved phases, however, do not behave the same way under decompression. Care must be exercised in applying model equations to each component. In the presence of increasing proportions of free phases, dissolved gas equations cannot track either species accurately.

Computational algorithms tracking both dissolved and free phases offer broader perspectives and expeditious alternatives, but with some changes from classical schemes. Free and dissolved gas dynamics differ. The *gradient* for free phase elimination increases with depth, directly opposite to the dissolved phase elimination gradient which decreases with depth. Then, changes in operational procedures become necessary for optimality. Impacts of this on decompression diving can be seen clearly in Figure 4, which contrasts supersaturation staging (USN and RN) against thermodynamic staging according to Hills. Similar profiles are seen in bubble models, such as the varying permeability approach of Yount and Hoffman. Considerations of excitation and growth invariably require deeper staging procedures than supersaturation methods. Though not as dramatic, similar constraints remain operative in multi-exposures, that is, multi-level, repetitive, and multi day diving.

Other issues concerning time sequencing of symptoms impact computational algorithms. That bubble formation is a predisposing condition for decompression sickness is universally accepted. However, formation

Figure 4. Phase And Supersaturation Decompression Profiles.

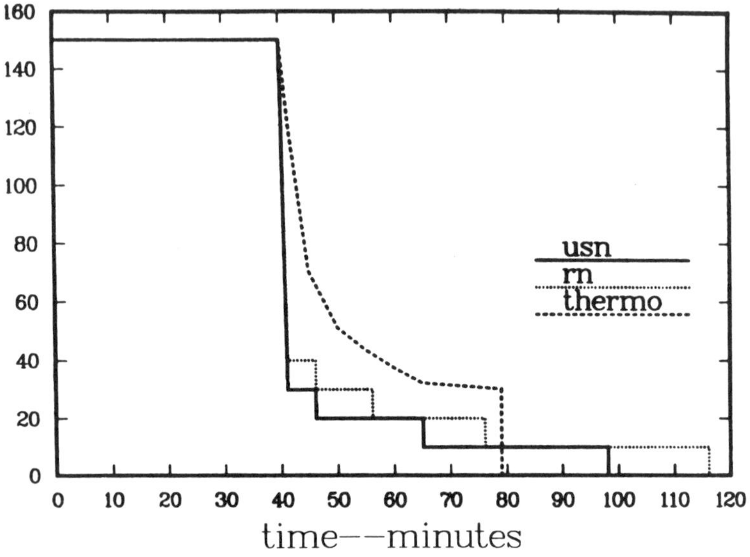

Decompression profiles for a dive to 150 fsw for 40 minutes are depicted according to supersaturation and critical phase formats. The supersaturation schedules (labeled USN and RN) obviously differ from the phase format (labeled thermo). Such differences are generic to bubble models versus critical tension models and involve:

1 — more time spent deeper to minimize bubble excitation and growth, and maximize the driving force to eliminate free phases, followed by;

2 — possible drop out at 20-30 fsw to dump asymptomatic free gas, if phase separation has been minimized by the overall ascent procedure.

Supersaturation formats with stops in the 10 to 30 fsw range might represent the treatment portion of the diving schedule, some believe. Computational analyses, some tests, and experiments have validated features of phase models, while work needs to continue on such approaches. Models extending biophysics can hopefully provide additional insights and optimal formats.

mechanisms and their ultimate physiological effect are two related, yet distinct, issues. On this point, most hypotheses make little distinction between bubble formation and the onset of bends symptoms. Yet we know that silent bubbles have been detected in subjects not suffering from decompression sickness. So it would thus appear that bubble formation, per se, and bends symptoms do not map onto each other in a one-to-one manner. Other factors are truly operative, such as the amount of gas dumped from solution, the size of nucleation sites receiving the gas, permissible bubble growth rates, deformation of surrounding tissue medium, and coalescence mechanisms for small bubbles into large aggregates, to name a few. These issues are the pervue of bubble theories, but the complexity of mechanisms addressed does not lend itself easily to table, nor even meter, implementation.

The ultimate computational algorithm, coupling nucleation, dissolved gas uptake and elimination, bubble growth and collisional coalescence, and critical sites, would be very, very complicated, requiring supercomputers (like CRAYs, CYBERs, VPs, CONVEXs, and ESSEXs, or their massively parallel cousins, CMs, NCUBESs, IWARPs, and DAPs) for three dimensional modeling. Stochastic Monte Carlo methods and sampling techniques exist which could generate and stabilize nuclei from thermodynamic functions, such as the Gibbs or Helmholtz free energy, transport dissolved gas in flowing blood to appropriate sites, inflate, deflate, move, and collide bubbles and nuclei, and then tally statistics on tensions, bubble size and number, inflation and coalescence rate, free phase volume, and any other meaningful parameter, all in necessary geometries. Such type simulations of similarly complicated problems last for 16-32 *hrs* at the Los Alamos and Livermore National Laboratories, on lightning fast supercomputers with near *gigaflop* speed (10^9 *floating point operations per second*). While decompression meters have revolutionized diving and decompression calculations, it will be some time before the ultimate computational algorithm fits into a wrist computer.

5.4. SLOW TISSUE COMPARTMENTS

Based on concerns in multi-day and heavy repetitive diving, with the hope of controlling staircasing gas buildup in exposures through critical tensions, slow tissue compartments ($\tau > 120$ *minutes*) have been incorporated into some algorithms. Calculations, however, show that virtually impossible exposures are required of the diver before critical tensions are even approached, literally tens of hours of near continuous activity. As noted in many calculations, slow compartments cannot really control multi-diving through critical tensions, unless critical tensions are reduced to absurd levels, inconsistent with non-stop time limits for shallow exposures. That is a model limitation, not necessarily a physical reality. The physical reality is that bubbles in slow tissues could be eliminated over time scales of days, and the model limitation is that the arbitrary parameter space does not accommodate such phenomena.

And that is no surprise either, when one considers that dissolved gas models are not supposed to track bubbles and free phases. Repetitive exposures do provide fresh dissolved gas for excited nuclei and growing free phases, but it is not the dissolved gas which is the problem just by itself. When bubble growth is considered, the slow compartments appear very important, because, therein, growing free phases are mostly left undisturbed insofar as surrounding tissue tensions are concerned. Bubbles grow more gradually in slow compartments because the gradient there is typically small, yet grow over longer time scales. When coupled to free phase dynamics, slow compartments are necessary in multi-diving calculations. The point is discussed further under free phase models.

For additional perspective, it should be noted that slow compartments have always been important in decompression and saturation diving, and flying-after-diving protocols. It is not clear now to what extent slow compartments are important to multi-diving. As testing continues, that should become clearer in the near future. But, based on inert gas washout experiments, some physiologists suggest that tissue compartments with half-lives near 720 *minutes* are to be found in bone, and possibly other sites. And bubbles have been found in subjects as long as three days after diving exposures. So, caution is the signal and models insensitive to slow compartments are limited at best.

5.5 VENOUS GAS EMBOLI

Sound reflected off a moving boundary undergoes a shift in acoustical frequency, the so-called Doppler shift. The shift is directly proportional to the speed of the moving surface (component in the direction of sound propogation) and the acoustical frequency of the wave, and inversely proportional to the sound speed. Acoustical signals in the *megahertz* range, termed ultrasound, have been directed at moving blood in the pulmonary arteries, where blood flow rates are the highest (near 20 *cm/sec*) due to confluence of the systemic circulation, with resulting Doppler shifts, in the form of audible chirps, snaps, whistles, and pops, noted and recorded. Sounds heard in divers have been ascribed to venous gas emboli (VGE), and *in vitro* simulations and evaluations have established minimum bubble detection size as a function of blood velocity. Coalesced lipids, platelet aggregates, and agglutinated red blood cells formed during decompression also pass through the pulmonary circulation, but are less reflective than bubbles, and usually smaller. Bubbles with radii in the 20 *micron* range represent a cut-off for Doppler detection for signals of a few *megahertz*.

Ultrasonic techniques for monitoring moving gas emboli in the pulmonary circulation are popular today. Silent bubbles, as applied to the venous gas emboli detected in sheep undergoing bends-free USN table decompression by Spencer and Campbell, were a first indication that asymptomatic free phases were present in blood, even under bounce loadings. Similar results were reported by Walder and Evans. After observing and contrasting venous gas emboli counts for various non-stop exposures at depth, Spencer suggested that non-stop limits be reduced below the USN table limits. Enforcing a 20% drop in venous gas emboli counts compared to the USN limits, corresponding non-stop limits, t_s, satisfy a reduced Hempleman relationship, that is, $dt_s^{1/2} = 465$ *fsw* min$^{1/2}$. Plugging those non-stop limits into the Haldane tissue equations for all depths and across all compartments, followed by extraction of the maximum of ensuing computed tissue tensions, permits construction of a reduced set of limiting tensions for table or meter implementation. Such exercises are quite popular today, and certainly prudent.

While the numbers of venous gas emboli detected with ultrasound Doppler techniques can be correlated with non-stop limits, and the limits then used to fine tune the critical tension matrix for select exposure ranges, fundamental issues are not necesarily resolved by venous gas emboli measurements. First of all, venous gas emboli are probably not the direct cause of bends per se, unless they block the pulmonary circulation, or pass through the pulmonary traps and enter the arterial system to lodge in critical sites. Intravascular bubbles might first form at extravascular sites. According to Hills, electron micrographs have highlighted bubbles breaking into capillary walls from adjacent lipid tissue beds in mice. Fatty tissue, draining the veins and possessing few nerve endings, is thought to be an extravascular site of venous gas emboli. Similarly, since blood constitutes no more than 8% of the total body capacity for dissolved gas, the bulk of circulating blood does not account for the amount of gas detected as venous gas emboli. Secondly, what has not been established is the link between venous gas emboli, possible micronuclei, and bubbles in critical tissues. Any such correlations of venous gas emboli with tissue micronuclei would unquestionably require considerable first-hand knowledge of nuclei size distributions, sites, and tissue thermodynamic properties. While some believe that venous gas emboli correlate with bubbles in extravascular sites, such as tendons and ligaments, and that venous gas emboli measurements can be reliably applied to bounce diving, the correlations with repetitive and saturation diving have not been made to work, nor important correlations with more severe forms of decompression sickness, such as chokes and central nervous system (CNS) hits.

Still, whatever the origin of venous gas emboli, procedures and protocols which reduce gas phases in the venous circulation deserve attention, for that matter, anywhere else in the body. The moving Doppler bubble may not be the bends bubble, but perhaps the difference may only be the present site. The propensity of venous gas emboli may reflect the state of critical tissues where decompression sickness does occur. Studies and tests based on Doppler detection of venous gas emboli are still the only viable means of monitoring free phases in the body. With that in mind, it is now sensible to consider another bends trigger point, the *critical volume* of separated gas, instead of the critical tension. The introduction of the concept by Hennessy and Hempleman has considerably impacted modern decompression modeling and analyses.

5.6 CRITICAL VOLUMES

In elegant experiments, Crocker and Goodenough exposed goats to compressed air at one absolute pressure, Q, for 12 hours (saturation) and then decompressed the animals to another absolute pressure, P, for several hours, checking for bends development. A few days later, the same animals were exposed to the same pressure, Q, and decompressed to slightly higher or lower pressure, P, until a distribution of P, separating bends from no-bends points, was generated. The whole *titration* was then repeated for a new series of Q. Repetitive exposures are, of course, not included in the titration.

Analyzing this data, and others from Gray and Masland, Hills proposed a complete separation of bends from no-bends points via a linear relationship between Q and P, redrawn in Figure 5 over the appropriate range, $0 < P < 200$ *fsw*. Similar type constraint curves are demonstrable for saturation diving at great depth. Over comparable pressure range, an interpolation between critical tensions and the titration curve is desirable to bridge saturation and bounce diving, but for given critical tension, only one tissue correlation could be established. This correlation is usually enforced in the slowest tissue compartment, like the 120 *minute* compartment in the Workman (USN) tables, and the 635 *minute* compartment in the Buhlmann (Swiss) tables, compartments controlling both saturation and repetitive diving. Obviously, any extrapolation from many bounce curves to just one curve for repetitive diving will be abrupt. Because of the linearity of the titration curve, it is also obvious that a constant decompression ratio, R, does not hold for saturation diving, that is, $R = M/P \neq constant$. Addressing these issues, Hills, and Hennessy and Hempleman proposed a working hypothesis, namely that after exposures to higher pressures, there are gaseous bubbles in tissues, and that the volume of this released gas is responsible for the onset of marginal symptoms of decompression sickness. The concept has proven useful in phase modeling and will be described, particularly with respect to bubble numbers and phase inflation rate.

Hennessy and Hempleman, and later Yount and Hoffman, established a linear titration curve for the data assuming that the same critical volume of released gas provokes mild attacks of decompression sickness. Such analyses also offer explanations for changes in signs and symptoms which follow changes in the nature of the exposure to pressure. Findings question and press dissolved gas approaches. While the titration experiment is compatible

Figure 5. Decompression Titration.

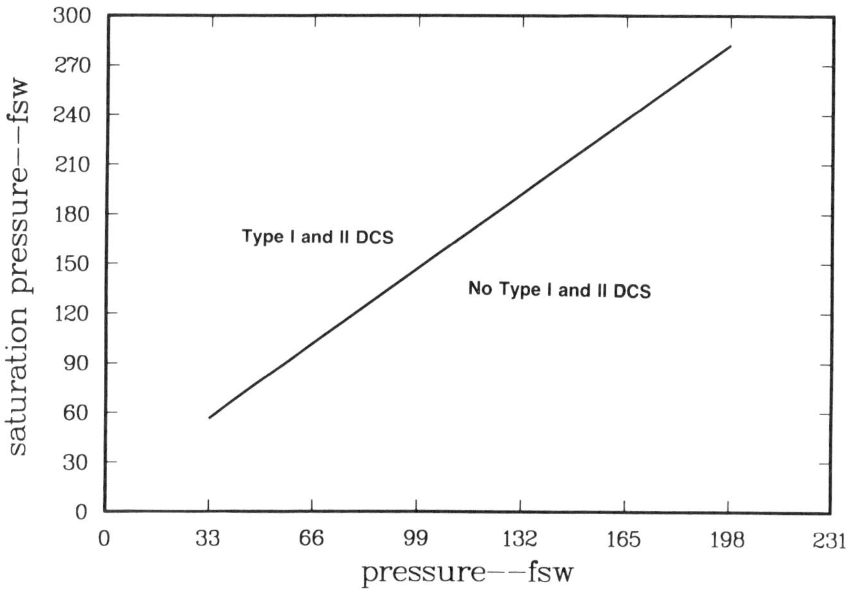

For simple bends (Type I and II), decompression titrations have been performed. A linear relationship between the saturation pressure, $Q = M/.79$, and permissible decompression, P, has been established over a range of exposures to depths less than 300 fsw. While predictions of critical tension models are close to the curve, only one compartment can match the curve. Models employing critical volumes recover the features (slope and intercept). The line is of the approximate form (fsw),

$$Q = 1.37\, P + 11.01,$$

according to Hills, Hennessy and Hempleman, and Yount and Hoffman. Most sets of table and meter algorithms recover the limiting form of the titration line in their slowest tissue compartments, that is critical tensions in the slowest compartment satisfy the above equation. The slowest compartments in most tables are also employed to restrict repetitive and multi-day exposures. Beyond 300 fsw the relationship becomes curvilinear. The original Haldane assignment of the same critical tension to all compartments is consistent with the titration experiment. One notes, however, that repetitive exposures are not cases in point here. In contrasting Figures 1a and 5, it is apparent that the body tolerates greater degrees of supersaturation and possibly more bubbles on short exposures than on longer exposures. The curve also shows that constant ratio, R, extrapolations do not hold for saturation diving.

with broad trends, it is clear that dissolved gas limiters, such as tensions, are often not the best critical flags. Indicators such as the volume fraction of separated gas are not only more natural, but are also more strongly correlated with experiment. Computational algorithms, coupling phase equilibration criteria or observed numbers of micronuclei in decompressed media to critical volumes, offer alternatives to the matrix of critical tensions. Fewer arbitrary parameters attend such treatments. The critical volume hypothesis also extends to mixed gases.

CHAPTER 6

Nucleation and Bubbles

Safety stops and slower ascent rates, in the context of dissolved gas models, are consistent with bubble mechanics, actually reducing bubble growth rate and free gas buildup because of greater effective pressure at the end of the dive. That is strong endorsement for the practice. Additionally, some regard safety stops, slower ascent rates, and increased off-gassing pressures as consistent treatment for separated (free) gas phases, particularly near the surface where further pressure reduction enhances growth. And gas nucleation theory and experiment tell us that on any given dive (compression-decompression), families of micronuclei larger than a critical (minimum) size are excited into bubble growth, so we must pay attention to free phase development throughout the dive. Experiments and calculations suggest that shallow, short stops and slow ascent rates have beneficial impact on reducing free phase buildup, while also reducing dissolved gas in the faster tissues. And that is important for deeper diving. Reasons are rooted ultimately in nucleation and bubble mechanics.

6.1 PHASE MECHANICS

Internal pressures in bubbles exceed ambient pressures by amounts equal to the effective surface tensions of the bubbles, as seen in Figure 6a. To eliminate bubbles, or reduce growth, *increasing* ambient pressure is requisite not only to restrict size, but also to drive the gas by diffusion out of the bubble and across the tissue-bubble interface, according to Figure 6b. The shorter the desired time of elimination, the greater must be the ambient pressure. Experiments conducted in decompressed gels, notably by Yount and Strauss, Kunkle and Beckman, and Yount, Yeung, and Gillary collectively, have been illuminating, testifying to the fact, as seen in Figure 7. The

Figure 6a. Bubble Pressure Balance.

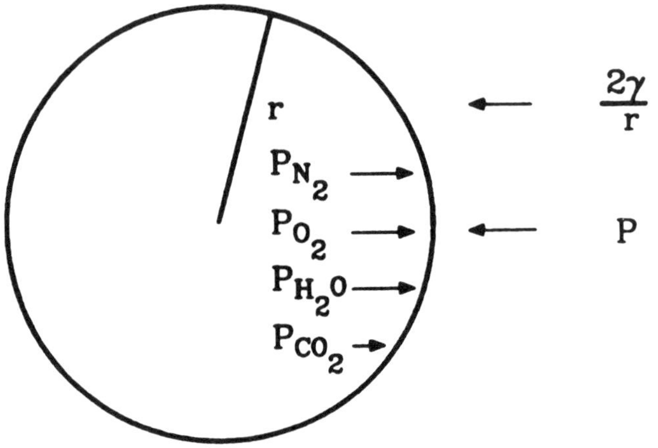

The total gas pressure, P_t, within an air bubble equals the sum of ambient pressure, P, plus effective surface tension, $2\gamma / r$, according to,

$$P_t = P + \frac{2\gamma}{r},$$

$$P_t = P_{O_2} + P_{N_2} + P_{H_2O} = P_{CO_2}.$$

At small radii, surface tension effects are large, while at large radii effects of surface tension vanish. Effective surface tension is the difference between Laplacian (thin film) tension and skin (surfactant) tension. Stabilized nuclei exhibit zero effective surface tension, so that total gas pressures and tensions are equal. When nuclei are destabilized (bubbles), any gradients between free and dissolved gas phases will drive the system to different configurations, that is, expansion or contraction, until a new equilibrium is established.

smaller the bubble, the shorter the dissolution time. Here implication for diving is rather clear. In the presence of even asymptomatic free phases, increased off-gassing pressure is prudent. With any pressure, the length of time required to dissolve bubbles of 250 *micron* diameter is significantly shorter than that required to dissolve larger bubbles. Immediate recompression within less than 5 *minutes* is adequate treatment for bubbles less than 100 *microns* in diameter, and forms the basis for Hawaiian and Australian emergency in-water recompression procedures. Such facts prop arguments

Figure 6b. Bubble Gas Diffusion.

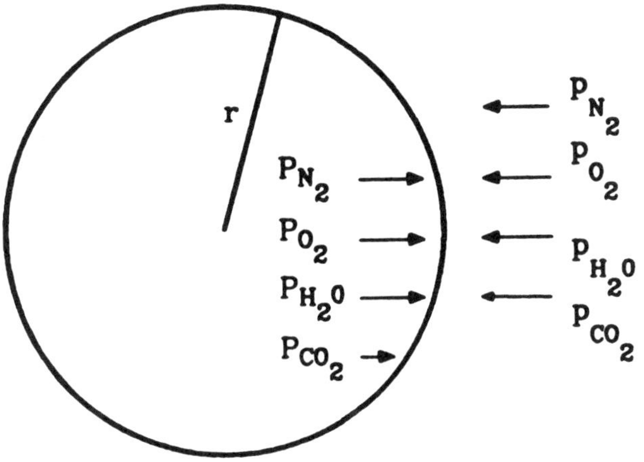

An air bubble in hydrostatic equilibrium will grow or contract, depending on its size and any relative gradients between free gas in the bubble and dissolved gas in tissue. Gradients are inward if tensions exceed bubble gas pressures, and outward if free gas pressures exceed tensions. A critical radius, r_c, separates growing from contracting bubbles for a given set of pressures. The critical radius depends on the total tension, p_t, ambient pressure, P, and effective surface tension, γ,

$$r_c = \frac{2\gamma}{p_t - P},$$

$$p_t = P_{N_2} + P_{O_2} + P_{H_2O} + P_{CO_2},$$

where growth occurs for $r > r_c$, and contraction for $r < r_c$. Some stabilized gas micronuclei in the body can always be excited into growth by pressure changes (compression-decompression).

for safety stops when conventional tables are pushed to limits, timewise or repetitively, assuming that gel and tissue bubbles respond to pressure in much the same manner.

Bubbles, which are unstable, might grow from micron size, gas nuclei which resist collapse due to elastic skins of surface-activated molecules (surfactants), or possibly reduction in surface tension at tissue interfaces or crevices. If families of these micronuclei persist, they vary in size and surfactant content. Large pressures (somewhere near 10 *atm*) are necessary to crush them. Micronuclei theoretically are small enough to pass through the

Figure 7. Dissolution Times for Graded Bubbles.

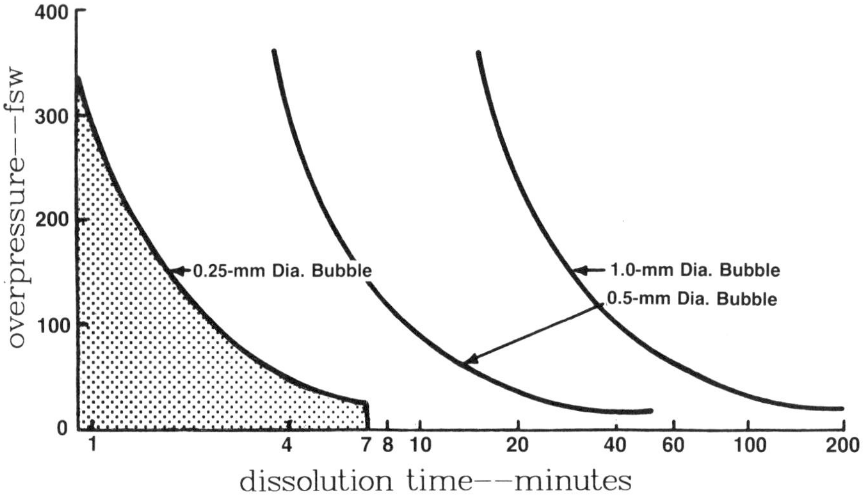

Bubbles develop and grow over longer time scales than nuclear stabilization. Yet, the rapid dissolution of bubbles in decompressed saturated gelatin (and the body proper) requires immediate and adequate repressurization. The absolute length of time required to dissolve bubbles with given overpressure is directly proportional to the size of the bubble. Obviously, the smaller the bubble, the shorter the time needed to dissolve that bubble at any overpressure. The bubbles studied in this experiment by Kunkle and Beckman grew to approximately 1 mm in 5 hrs, starting from stabilized micronuclei. Such experiments have provided vital information, corroborating nucleation and bubble theories in vitro.

pulmonary filters, yet dense enough not to float to the surfaces of their environments, with which they are in both hydrostatic (pressure) and diffusion (gas flow) equilibrium. When nuclei are stabilized, and not activated to growth or contraction by external pressure changes, the skin (surfactant) tension offsets both the Laplacian (film) tension and any mechanical help from surrounding tissue. Then all pressure and gas tensions are equal. However, on decompression, the seed pockets are surrounded by dissolved gases at high tension and can subsequently grow (bubbles) as surrounding gas diffuses into them. The rate at which bubbles grow, or contract, depends directly on the difference between tissue tension and local ambient pressure, effectively the bubble pressure gradient, denoted G. At some point in time, a critical volume of bubbles, or separated gas, is established and bends symptoms become statistically more probable. On compression, the micronuclei are crunched down to smaller sizes across families, apparently stabilizing at new reduced size. Bubbles are also crunched by increasing pressure because of Boyle's law, and then additionally shrink if gas diffuses out of them. As bubbles get smaller and smaller, they possibly restabilize as micronuclei.

Under compression-decompression, gas nuclei may grow as bubbles, depending on their effective surface tension and bubble radius. Below a certain critical radius, listed in Table 3 as a function of pressure according to the varying permeability model (VPM), bubbles tend to collapse on themselves, while at larger equilibrium radius, they grow as gas diffuses into them. Stabilized nuclei evolve into unstable bubbles when their effective surface tension is greater than zero, or a sufficient diffusion gradient exists to drive gas into or out of the nucleus. At sea level, the excitation radius is near .8 *microns*, smaller than living cells, having dimensions starting at a few microns.

Table 3. Micronuclei Excitation Radii.

pressure *P (fsw)*	excitation radius *r (microns)*	pressure *P (fsw)*	excitation radius *r (microns)*
13	.89	153	.49
33	.80	173	.46
53	.72	193	.44
73	.66	213	.41
93	.61	233	.39
113	.57	253	.37
133	.53	273	.36

Nucleation theory is consistent with a number of diving observations. Divers can significantly increase tolerance against bubble formation, and therefore bends, by following three simple practices, originally suggested by Walder, Evans and Walder, Albano and Griscuoli, and reiterated by Yount, Kunkle, and Beckman:

(1) make the first dive a deep, short (crush) dive, thereby constricting micronuclei down to smaller, safer size;
(2) make succeeding dives progressively more shallow, thus diving within crush limits of the first dive and minimizing excitation of smaller micronuclei; and,
(3) make frequent dives (like every other day), thus depleting the number of micronuclei available to form troublesome bubbles.

An underlying point can be made here. If nucleation sites are extinguished, reduced in number, or ill-disposed to excitation, bubble formation and risk are commensurately reduced. Regeneration times for classes of micronuclei are estimated to be near a week, underscoring physiological adaptation to recurring pressure environments. The mechanics of nucleation, stabilization, and bubble growth are fairly complex, with stabilization mechanisms only recently quantified. Source and generation mechanisms before stabilization are not well understood. Some candidates include cosmic radiation and charged particles, dissolved gases in fluids we drink, lymph draining tissues into veins, collisional coalescence, blood turbulence and vorticity, exercise, the stomach, and the thin air-blood endothelium in the lungs. Once formed, micronuclei must stabilize very rapidly with surfactant material. Passing through the pulmonary filters to the lungs, only submicron sizes might survive. If nuclei are persistent, it is not clear that they populate all tissue sites, nor possess the same size distributions. Some can argue that gel findings are not relevant because biological fluids are formed, and contained, in a sealed environment (the body), but the Strauss and Yount studies confirm the existence of preformed gas micronuclei in blood serum and egg albumin. Nuclei seem to pervade all manner of fluids.

Abandoning preformed nuclei, other methods of bubble formation are certainly possible. Cavitation, produced by the rapid tearing or moving apart of tissues interfaces, is a candidate, as well as surface friction (tribonucleation). Crevices in tissues may form or trap gas phases, with later potential for release. Vorticity in blood flow patterns might cause small microbubbles. Stable, or unstable, the copious presence of microbubbles in the venous circulation would impact dissolved gas elimination adversely, also possibly impairing the lungs or the arterial network. The presence of bubbles in the arterial circulation might result in embolism. Bubble clogging of the pulmonary circulation is thought to relate to the *chokes*, a serious form of decompression sickness, while cerebral decompression sickness is believed due to emboli. Microbubbles in the venous circulation would render gas uptake and elimination asymmetric, with uptake faster than elimination. Displacing blood, microbubbles would reduce the effective area and volume for tissue-blood gas exchange.

6.2 SURFACTANTS

Water, gasoline, glycerin, and salad oil are clearly liquids. Pancake syrup, paste, egg white, silly putty, paint, glue, and dishwashing soap are also liquids, that is, they flow on the application of stress, but border on scientific classification on all other grounds. In all mechanical response, but particularly viscosity, the latter class differs from each other as much as they differ from solids. And the response is variable in time. Syrup becomes sticky as it dries. Dishwashing soap often dries into light flakes. Silly putty flows on tilt, but shatters on sudden impact. Airplane glue is springy and rubbery.

Substances in the latter list are called structured fluids, owing their distinctive and unusual properties to large, polyatomic structures, many times the size of a water molecule. Fluids containing polyatomic structures manifest a wide variety of mechanical response and self-organization. Body tissues and fluids host an uncountable collection of both organic and inorganic matter, with many biochemical substances falling into the structured fluid category. Among those structured fluids, a class of self-assemblies, called surfactants, are very interesting, possessing properties which can stabilize microbubbles in various stages of evolution by offsetting surface tension.

A surfactant is a structured fluid which is *ambiphilic,* incorporating parts that assume preferential orientations at water-oil (immiscible) interfaces. A surfactant molecule usually consists of a bulky ion at one head, and a counterion at the tail. Isolated molecules cannot usually exist in one media type, or another, but instead orient themselves into *micelles*, configurations in which like parts clump together, that is, head in one substance and tail in the other. Micelles typically have diameters on the order of 10^{-3} *microns*, and render the interfaces unlike anything measured in the components. Lipid-aquaeous tissue interfaces potentially present favorable environments for surfactants.

In certain conditions, a surfactant can reduce interfacial surface tension, allowing the interface to grow and wrap around itself. The result is a microbundle full of alternating interfaces, spherical in structure to minimize thermodynamic energy constraints. Many substances may be bound up in the microbundle. If small gas nuclei, but typically much larger than a micelle, are in contact with the interfaces, or surfactants directly, a spherical gas micronucleus-microemulsion might develop, varying in size and surfactant content. The assembly is stable when the effective surface tension is zero, when surfactant skin pressure just balances mechanical (Laplace) surface tension. If the effective surface tension of the nucleus, γ, is not zero, the collection will grow or contract until stable, or disassemble. In the case of gas microemulsions, the surfactant is thought to coat the inside boundary layer mostly, with the free gas in the interior. The actual configuration is probably more complex, but such a picture can be drawn for simplicity in calculations. Surfactant stabilized micronuclei may theoretically destabilize under compression-decompression processes in diving, perhaps spawning bubble growth fueled by high gas tension in surrounding media. Microbubbles may remain localized at the interfaces, but probably migrate. Sources of initial gas nuclei, surfactant compositions, and tissue sites await description.

6.3 EMPIRICAL PRACTICES

Utilitarian procedures, entirely consistent with phase mechanics and bubble dissolution time scales, have been developed under duress, and with trauma, by Australian pearl divers and Hawaiian diving fishermen, for both deep and repetitive diving with possible in-water recompression for hits. While the science behind such procedures was not initially clear, the operational effectiveness was always noteworthy and could not be discounted easily. Later, the rationale, essentially recounted in the foregoing, became clearer.

Pearling fleets, operating in the deep tidal waters off northern Australia, employed Okinawan divers who regularly journeyed to depths of 300 *fsw* for as long as one hour, two times a day, six days per week, and ten months out of the year. Driven by economics, and not science, these divers developed optimized decompression schedules empirically. As reported by LeMessurier and Hills, deeper decompression stops, but shorter decompression times than required by Haldane theory, were characteristics of their profiles. Such protocols are entirely consistent with minimizing bubble growth and the excitation of nuclei through the application of increased pressure, as are shallow safety stops and slow ascent rates. With higher incidence of surface decompression sickness, as might be expected, the Australians devised a simple, but very effective, in-water recompression procedure. The stricken diver is taken back down to 30 *fsw* on oxygen for roughly 30 *minutes* in mild cases, or 60 *minutes* in severe cases. Increased pressures help to constrict bubbles, while breathing pure oxygen maximizes inert gas washout (elimination). Recompression time scales are consistent with bubble dissolution experiments.

Similar schedules and procedures have evolved in Hawaii, among diving fishermen, according to Farm and Hayashi. Harvesting the oceans for food and profit, Hawaiian divers make between 8 and 12 dives a day to depths beyond 350 *fsw*. Profit incentives induce divers to take risks relative to bottom time in conventional tables. Three repetitive dives are usually necessary to net a school of fish. Consistent with bubble and nucleation theory, these divers make their deep dive first, followed by shallower excursions. A typical series might start with a dive to 220 *fsw*, followed by 2 dives to 120 *fsw*, and culminate in 3 or 4 more excursions to less than 60 *fsw*. Often, very short or zero surface intervals are clocked between dives. Such types of profiles literally clobber conventional tables, but, with proper reckoning of bubble and phase mechanics, acquire some credibility. With ascending profiles and suitable application of pressure, gas seed excitation and any bubble growth are constrained within the body's capacity to eliminate free and dissolved gas phases. In a broad sense, the final shallow dives have been tagged as prolonged safety stops, and the effectiveness of these procedures has been substantiated *in vivo* (dogs) by Kunkle and Beckman. In-water recompression procedures, similar to the Australian regimens, complement Hawaiian diving practices for all the same reasons.

While the above practices developed by trial-and-error, albeit with seeming principle, venous gas emboli measurements, performed off Catalina by

Figure 8a. Reduction In VGE Counts Following Safety Stops.

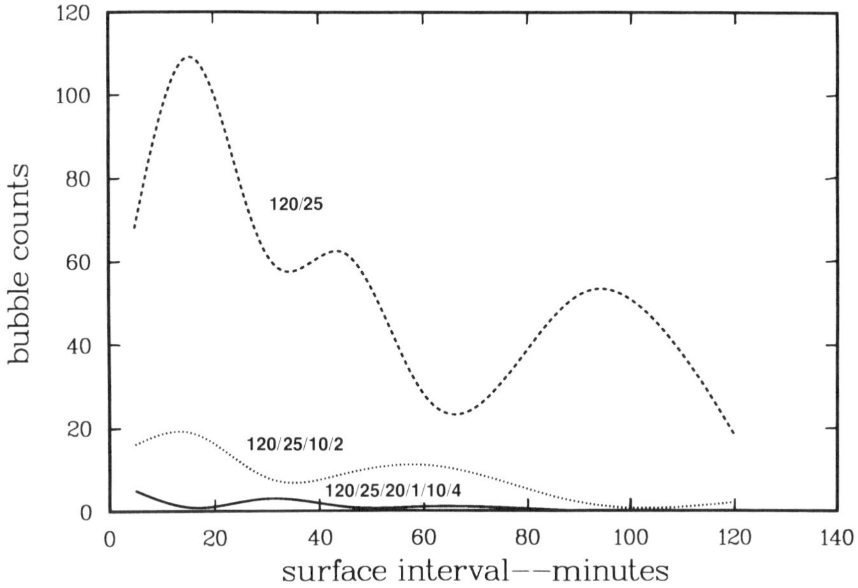

Safety stops have considerable impact on Doppler sounded VGE measurements, according to Pilmanis. Following a dive to 100 fsw for 25 minutes, the top curve registers VGE counts over increasing surface interval time. The lower two curves depict the count after a brief stop for 2 minutes at 10 fsw, and then 1 minute at 20 fsw followed by 4 minutes at 10 fsw. Reductions by factors of 4-6 are apparent. Whether VGE correlate with susceptibility to DCS, or not, free phase reduction in the pulmonary circulation is impressive with shallow safety stops.

Pilmanis on divers making shallow safety stops, fall into the more *scientific* category perhaps. Contrasting bubble counts following bounce exposures near 100 *fsw*, with and without zonal stops in the 10-20 *fsw* range, marked reductions (factors of 4 to 5) in venous gas emboli, as seen in Figure 8a, were noted when stops were made. If, as some suggest, venous gas emboli in bounce diving correlate with bubbles in sites such as tendons and ligaments, then safety stops probably minimize bubble growth in such extravascular locations. In these tests, the sample population was small, so additional validation and testing is warranted.

6.4. STOPS AND ASCENT RATES

Attempts to track free phases within patently dissolved phase models may not optimize, but still can be mocked up for consistency with phase dynamics. One approach is to slow ascent rates and/or introduce safety

Figure 8b. Bubble Growth With Varying Ascent Rate.

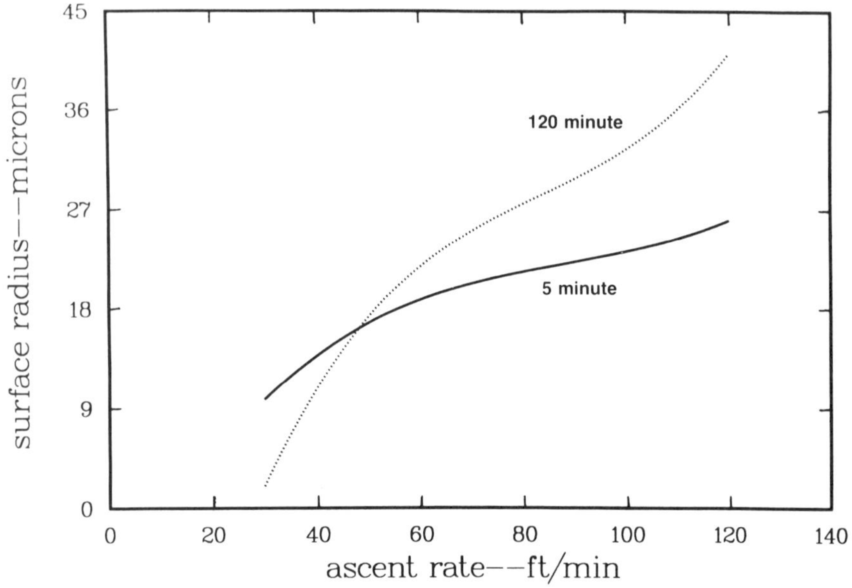

The rate at which bubbles grow on ascent depends on their size and surface tension, and the average difference between tissue tension and ambient pressure. For bubbles larger than a certain critical (cutoff) radius, faster ascents in the presence of elevated gas tensions in surrounding tissue sites tend to support growth, because average ambient pressure, P, is lessened by fast ascent. Increasing ambient pressure always tends to restrict simple bubble growth, since internal bubble pressure is always greater than ambient pressure by an amount, $2\gamma/r$. In this calculation, $2\gamma = 8.3$ fsw micron, and unit solubility, concentration, and diffusivity employed for simplicity. One notes that the growth rate in the 5 minute compartment is less than in the 120 minute compartment. Ostensibly the faster compartment off-gases more rapidly during any ascent, presenting a lower average tension and weaker diffusion gradient for growth.

stops strategically. As far as net gas exchange is concerned, most combinations of stops and rates can be equivalenced to almost any other set at given pressure, so there is always some leeway. Growth minimization and free phase elimination favor slow ascents. Figure 8b plots surfacing radius of an initially small bubble *($r = .36$ microns)*, held in both fast and slow tissue compartments, as a function of ascent rate. The results are typical for classes of bounce and repetitive diving, and underscore growth minimization with slow ascent rate due to increased ambient pressure on the average.

Based on suggestions at an American Academy Of Underwater Sciences ascent workshop, recorded by Lang and Egstrom, discretionary safety stops for 2-4 *minutes* in the 10-20 *fsw* zone are recommended. Calculations reported by Wienke, Hamilton, and Lewis, and summarized in Tables 4a and 4b, underscore the bases of the suggestions for a number of reasons. Relative changes in three computed trigger points, tissue tension, separated phase volume, and bubble radius, are listed for six compartments following a nominal bounce dive to 120 *fsw* for 12 *minutes*, with and without a safety stop at 15 *fsw* for 3 *minutes*. Stop procedures markedly restrict bubble and phase volume growth, while permitting insignificant levels of dissolved gas buildup in the slow tissues. The reduction in growth parameters far outstrips any dissolved gas buildup in slow compartments, and faster compartments naturally eliminate dissolved gases during the stop, important for deeper diving.

Table 4a. Relative Changes In Critical Parameters After Safety Stop.

τ *(min)* half-life	tissue tension relative change	critical volume relative change	bubble radius relative change
5	-21%	-34%	-68%
10	-11%	-24%	-39%
20	-6%	-11%	-24%
40	-2%	-8%	-18%
80	1%	3%	-2%
120	2%	4%	1%

Safety stop time can be added to bottom time for additional conservatism, but the effect of neglecting stop time is also small, as seen in Table 4b. A stop at 15 *fsw* for 2 *minutes* is roughly equivalent to more than halving the standard ascent rate at depths in excess of 120 *fsw*. Procedures such as this, as well as reduced no-stop time limits, appear beneficial in multi-day, multi-level, and repetitive diving. A safety stop near 15 *fsw* is easier than 10 *fsw* in adverse water conditions, such as surge and surface disturbances. Slower ascent rates afford additional advantages, but safety stops in the 2-4 *minute* range are easier and more efficient.

Table 4b. Comparative Surfacing Tissue Tensions.

τ *(min)* half-life	surfacing tension *(fsw)* 120 *fsw*/15 min	surfacing tension *(fsw)* 120 *fsw*/12 min 15 *fsw*/3 min	surfacing tension *(fsw)* 120 *fsw*/15 min 15 *fsw*/3 min
5	101.5	77.0	79.7
10	87.5	73.0	78.1
20	66.9	59.0	64.0
40	49.9	45.7	49.2
80	39.0	36.9	38.9
120	34.9	33.5	34.8

At altitude the same procedures can be employed, with depths, ascent rates, and stops conservatively scaled by the altitude correction factors (ratio of sea level pressure to ambient pressure at altitude) when using tables for which critical tensions need extrapolation at reduced ambient pressure. Tables with critical tensions fitted to altitude data have their own rules, as do meters.

Generally, bubble growth and excitation are compounded at altitude because of reduced pressure. The modeling work of Van Liew, Gernhardt and Lambertsen underscores this fact, indicating why critical tension models often fall short in hypobaric applications. Bubbles grow faster as they get bigger, and as pressure drops. With decreased pressure, bubbles will also expand by Boyle's law. Bigger bubbles are not as constricted by Laplacian film tension, while reduced pressure supports a faster rate of tissue gas diffusion into the bubble itself. Lanphier and Lehner performed extensive aerial decompression studies with goats, concluding that aerial decompression sickness strongly resembles underwater decompression sickness following saturation exposure. For ranging profiles followed by decompression to ambient pressure, a high incidence of chokes was noted. Chokes is thought to result from microemboli interfering with pulmonary function. It is easy to speculate that rapid decompression to reduced pressure contributes to the buildup and growth of pulmonary emboli for the same reasons. Lanphier also concluded that slow tissue ($\tau \geq 80$ *minutes*) compartments do not correlate with chokes, suggesting that pulmonary microemboli are linked to fast compartments. Clearly, such an assertion also points out differences between types of decompression sickness, inferred critical tissue half-lives, and bubble formation time scales. Chokes and limb bends result from different critical insults, at different places, and over possibly different time scales.

The point to be made here in all cases is simple. Increased off-gassing pressures reduce bubble growth rates dramatically in shallow zones, while impacting dissolved gas buildup in the slowest compartments minimally. Fast compartments also off-load gas during safety stops, important for deep diving. Stops and slow ascent rates are always advisable, but particularly in multi-activities.

6.5. ACCLIMATIZATION

Divers and caisson workers have long contended that tolerance to decompression sickness increases with daily diving, and decreases after a few weeks layoff. Paton and Walder, Golding and Griffiths have confirmed such suggestions, pointing out that in large groups of compressed air workers, new workers were at higher risk than those who were exposed to high pressure regularly. This acclimatization might result from either increased body tolerance to bubbles (physiological adaption), or decreased number and volume of bubbles (physical adaptation). Walder advocated physical adaptation, resulting from systematic destruction or reduction in gas micronuclei, from which bubbles grow. Kunkle and Beckman monitored venous gas emboli in the pulmonary arteries of dogs, noting that the number of total emboli counted decreased as the repetitive frequency increased, but that the same bubble number precipitated decompression sickness in all cases. Repetitive spacings were on the order of a day or two in the experiments, and results are clearly consistent with physical adaptation.

Yet, there is another slight inconsistency here. Statistics point to higher bends incidence in repetitive and multi-day diving. Some hyperbaric specialists confirm the same, based on experience. The situation is not clear, but the resolution plausibly links to the kinds of first dives made and repetitive frequency in the sequence. If the first in a series of repetitive dives are kept short, deep, and conservative with respect to non-stop time limits, initial bubble excitation and growth are minimized. Subsequent dives would witness minimal levels of initial phases. If surface intervals are also long enough to optimize both free and dissolved gas elimination, any nuclei excited into growth could be efficiently eliminated outside repetitive exposures, with adaptation occuring over day intervals as noted in experiments. But higher frequency, repetitive and multi-day loading may not afford sufficient surface intervals to eliminate free phases excited by earlier exposures, with additional nuclei then possibly excited on top of existing phases. Physical adaptation seems less likely, and decompression sickness more likely, in the latter case. Daily regimens of a single bounce dive with slightly increasing exposure times are consistent with physical adaptation, and conservative practices. The regimens also require deepest dives first. In short, acclimatization is as much a question of eliminating any free phases formed as it is a question of crushing or reducing nuclei as potential bubbles in repetitive exposures. And then time scales on the order of a day might limit the adaptation process. The conservative repetitive protocols discussed are consistent with such reasoning, as are bubble models employing growth and elimination time constants on the same scale.

CHAPTER 7

Free Gas Phase Models

Previous tables for humans were based upon unsupported assumptions because many of the underlying processes by which dissolved gas is liberated from blood and tissues were poorly understood. Some of those assumptions, as enumerated by Hills and Yount, are now known to be wrong. Recent developments in bubble nucleation models, linked to experiments, have made it possible to calculate diving tables from more established principles. Both flexibility and range of applicability are impressive, and they recover dissolved gas models in the proper limits.

7.1 PHASE SEPARATION

Only a handful of hard and fast conclusions about simple decompression sickness can be drawn from our present knowledge. So elementary as to be innocuous, they can be stated:

(1) bubble inception or phase separation is the primary event triggering simple decompression sickness;
(2) prevention of decompression sickness amounts to prevention (as a limit) of bubble inception or phase separation; and
(3) gradual pressure reductions minimize bubble formation.

As pointed out by many, after the above statements, concensus usually diverges. Modelers and table designers must then supply or assume, gas exchange models, trigger points, and safe diving protocols which prevent, or at least minimize, phase inception and bubble growth.

Present notions of nucleation and cavitation suggest that decompression phase separation is random, yet highly probable, in body tissue. Once established, a gaseous phase will further grow by acquiring gas from adjacent saturated tissue, according to the strength of the free-dissolved gradient, as studied by Epstein and Plesset, Powell, Buckles, Nims, Bateman and Lang, Strauss, Yount, Kunkle, Van Liew and Bishop, Walder, Beckman, and Gernhardt and Lambertson. Although exchange mechanisms are better understood, nucleation and stabilization mechanisms remain less so, and calculationally elusive. Stochastic Monte Carlo bubble tracking methods are powerful, but only in supercomputer environments, due to the large number of events required for meaningful statistics over simulation time spans. Exchange models for entrained bubbles and coalescence dynamics are similarly complicated. In all cases, more knowledge about gas micronuclei and size distributions, tissue sites, thermodynamics properties, stabilization, and excitation mechanisms is necessary before computing power can be leveraged to decompression modeling.

But even with a paucity of earlier information, many feel that some of the recent studies on bubbles and nuclei shed considerable light on growth and elimination processes, and time scales. Their consistency with underlying physical principles suggest directions for table and meter modeling, beyond parameter fitting and extrapolation techniques. Recovering dissolved gas algorithms for short exposure times, phase models link to both bubble mechanics and critical volume trigger points.

7.2 VARYING PERMEABILITY MODEL

To evaluate and apply laboratory studies of bubble growth and nucleation in gels, Yount and Hoffman developed a comprehensive set of air tables, and compared them to the USN and RN conventional tables. Decompressions, bounce diving, altitude bends, and saturation diving are all successfully described by one setting of four global parameters, replacing the usual set of critical tensions. This set is remarkably self-consistent, permitting accurate interpolation and extrapolation. And this methodology is useful in extending the model to multi-diving.

The outcome of their studies has been the development of a varying permeability bubble model (VPM), described in Appendix D, in which cavitation nuclei of gas phases are small enough to remain in solution and strong enough to resist collapse, their stability provided by elastic skins or membranes consisting of surface-active molecules. Ordinarily, bubble skins are permeable to gas, but can become impermeable when subjected to large compressions (near 10 *atm*). By tracking the changes in nuclear radius that are caused by increases or decreases in ambient pressure, the varying permeability model provides precise quantitative descriptions of several bubble-counting experiments carried out in supersaturated gel. The model has also been used to trace levels of incidence of decompression sickness in animal species such as shrimp, salmon, rats, and humans. Microscopic evidence has also been obtained which indicates the spherical gas nuclei, those persistent microbubbles, actually do exist and possess physical properties consistent with earlier assignments. For example, nuclear radii are on the order of 1 *micron* or less, and their number density in bio-media decreases exponentially with increasing radius, characteristic of a system gas nuclei in equilibrium with their surroundings at the same temperature. While bubbles in the body are perfused and certainly subject to metabolic processes, the mechanics of compression-decompression for these bubbles is initially the same as gel bubbles. Time scales for growth and dissolution would then seem to be a difference between the two, controlled by the composition of the gas breathing mixture, relative component solubility, and diffusivity.

The primary bubbles formed directly from nuclei may lead to secondary bubbles via *fission* in the blood, or by the creation of *rosaries* in the interstitial spaces of firmer tissues. Since tissue deformation and impairment of circulation should depend upon both the size and number of bubbles, it seems plausible that the total volume of evolved gas would serve as an effective criteria in any bubble model. For short decompression times, bubble nuclei have little time to inflate. The permissible critical radius is then smaller, and the allowed supersaturation larger, resulting in many small bubbles. Conversely, during long decompressions, bubbles may grow very large, so that only a few are permitted. In the varying permeability model, it is thus assumed that the body is able to accommodate a certain number of *safe* bubbles for long periods of time. Compression-decompression will excite bubbles in excess of that safe number, denoted Δn, depending on depth and time. For short bounce dives, Δn can be large, while for saturation diving, Δn must be small.

Because the size distribution and number density of gas nuclei *in vivo* are unknown, the model uses an iterative procedure in algorithms. Under such circumstance, unknown parameters, usually minimal in number compared to the matrix of critical tensions, can be evaluated from small data sets and accurately used to extrapolate to other regimes. In the case of the varying permeability model, only five parameters are necessary. Interesting features, arising naturally within the model, include:

(1) reduced non-stop time limits;
(2) safety stops (or shallow swimming ascents) in the 10-20 *fsw* zone, 1-2 *minutes* for dives in the 40-90 *fsw* range, 2-3 *minutes* for dives in the 90-240 *fsw* range;
(3) ascent rates not exceeding 60 *fsw/min;*
(4) restricted repetitive exposures, particularly beyond 100 *fsw*, based on reduction in permissible bubble excess over time;
(5) restricted spike (shallow-to-deep) exposures based on excitation of additional micronuclei;

(6) restricted multi-day activity based on regeneration of micronuclei over longer time scales;
(7) smooth coalescence of bounce and saturation limit points, consistent with bubble experiments; and
(8) consistent model treatment of altitude diving.

Bubble models tend to be consistent with the earlier conservative measures suggested for diving practice. Conservatism may be downplayed in some meter implementations, yet medical authorities are becoming increasingly concerned about long term effects of breathing pressurized gases. On firmer principles, bubble models tend to corroborate safety measures in multi-diving, and thus one might reasonably expect to witness their further development. Said another way, bubble models have the right physical signatures for diving application.

7.3 CRITICAL GRADIENTS

Any set of non-stop time limits can be plugged into model equations, and maximum computed tensions across all compartments and depths assigned as limiting tensions, M, with corresponding critical gradients, G, obtained by subtracting ambient pressure, P, from absolute M, that is, $G = M/.79 - P$. Using the reduced time limits, listed in Table 5a, we can construct a conservative set of gradients for purposes of illustration and discussion. The bounce gradient, G_0, is first computed for each compartment, τ, across the half-life spectrum, $1 \leq \tau \leq 720$ *minutes*. Non-stop exposures, with direct surface ascent, thus allows G_0 for that compartment. Defining the relative change in gradient with depth ΔG, the full gradient, $G = G_0 + \Delta G d$, is defined for any exposure. Both G_0 and ΔG are tabulated in Table 5b, with ΔG, interpolated from Buhlmann and Workman. Time limits are conservative, so the gradients are also conservative. The extrapolation to altitude, that is, $d = P - 33$, is also implied in the algorithm.

Note that fast compartments at greater depths permit larger G, while slower compartments at shallower depth require smaller G, reflecting the body's ability to support increased degrees of supersaturation with increased pressure. Bubbles and micronuclei tend to both shrink and possibly stabilize under pressure, permitting increased levels of supersaturation because of greater surface tension. Under decompression, smaller bubbles and nuclei also grow more slowly for the same reason. Surface tension pressure, varying inversely as the spherical radius, r, helps to expel gas in the pocket by squeezing and building up a diffusion gradient across the film boundary. Unless nuclei are stabilized so that the net surface tension pressure is zero, all nuclei would eventually collapse upon themselves because of this squeeze. When nuclei are squeezed by increasing pressure, gel experiments established that they stabilize at new smaller radius, not growing back to earlier size unless ambient pressure is reduced. While gel is neither metabolic nor perfused, and processes in tissue must impact nucleation and bubble dynamics, pressure mechanics are similar. It is the physics we understand, but much less the physiology, of bubbles.

Table 5a. Bounce Time Limits.

depth *d (fsw)*	**time limit** t_s *(minutes)*	**depth** *d (fsw)*	**time limit** t_s *(minutes)*
10	1840	130	9.
20	483	140	8.
30	230	150	7.
40	108	160	6.
50	65	170	5.5
60	40	180	5.
70	30	190	4.5
80	24	200	4.
90	18	210	3.5
100	15	220	3.
110	13	230	2.6
120	11	240	2.3

Although the actual size distribution of gas nuclei in humans is unknown, the Yount and Kunkle experiments *in vitro* (gels) suggest a decaying exponential is reasonable. Under such circumstance, a larger number of small nuclei are excited into growth by deep decompressions, and a smaller number excited by shallow decompressions. Permissible bubble numbers, Δn, are also greater for short dives, and lesser for long dives. Both bubble excess, Δn, critical tension, M, and critical gradient, G, are coupled in application, with Δn tracking free phases and G dissolved phases. Their interaction drives the amount of separated phase volume, V_{crit}, the trigger point in bubble models. The phase volume changes under loading, just as tissue tension and bubble number. Long surface intervals permit reductions in tissue tensions, bubble numbers, and separated phase volumes. But, because the dynamics of elimination of free and dissolved gas phases differ, component elimination rates vary with surfacc interval, and the phase volumc, tracking as the product of the bubble number, Δn, and the gradient, G, changes in a complicated manner.

The rate at which gas inflates in tissue depends upon the product of bubble excess, Δn, and supersaturation gradient, G. The phase volume

Table 5b. Bounce Gradients.

half-life τ *(minutes)*	surface gradient G_0 *(fsw)*	gradient change ΔG
1	192	.519
2	150	.518
5	94	.515
10	65	.511
20	46	.506
40	34	.468
80	26	.417
120	22	.379
180	18	.354
240	16	.329
360	12	.321
480	11	.312
720	8	.303

hypothesis, quantified in Appendix D, constrains the sum of the product of the two over time to always remain less than some limit point, $\epsilon\ V_{crit}$, with ϵ a proportionality constant and V_{crit} the critical separated phase volume. The critical gradients then can be consistently extracted from $\epsilon\ V_{crit}$, r_0, and other related bubble constants. The approach is aptly called a bootstrap.

7.4 REDUCED GRADIENT BUBBLE MODEL

Extending the same phase hypothesis to multi-diving, Wienke has shown that any set of bounce gradients, G, like Table 5b, can be employed for repetitive diving, providing they are reduced to successive exposures, as sketched in Appendix E. The extension, coupled to the varying permeability model, is called the reduced gradient bubble model (RGBM). Denoting the reduced set, $\bar{G}$, we write symbolically, $\bar{G} = \xi\ G$, in terms of the bounce gradients G, for ξ a set of *multi-diving* fractions bounded in relative terms, that is, $0 \leq \xi \leq 1$. As repetitive time intervals decrease, appropriate ξ should get smaller and staging approach saturation limits. As repetitive time intervals increase, ξ should get larger, and staging approach bounce limits. In between total elapsed time, total surface interval, tissue compartment, and profile determine ξ. Considering interpolating behavior, a checklist of properties of ξ, correlating the model with diving practice is desirable:

(1) ξ equals one for a bounce dive, remaining less than one for repetitive dives within characteristic time;

Figure 9a. Repetitive Factors.

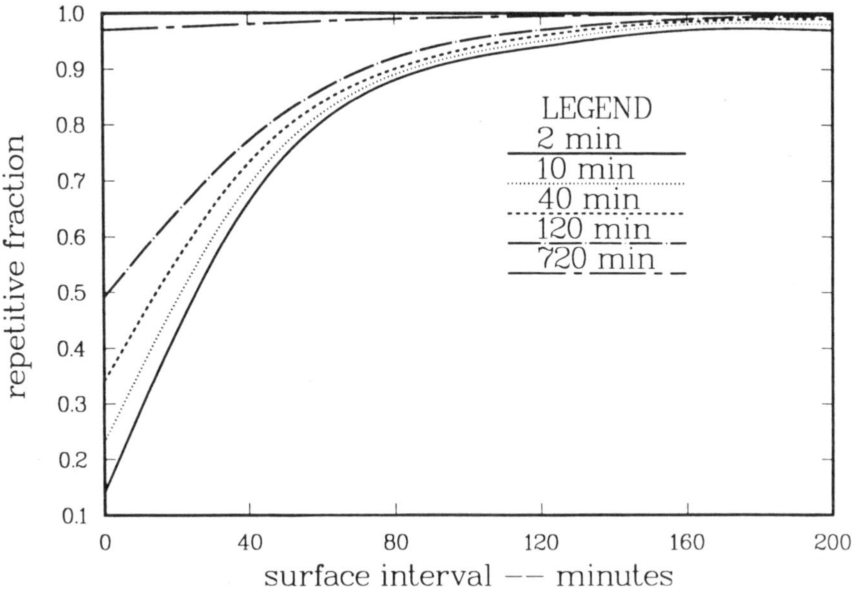

Within the phase volume constraint, bubble elimination periods are shortened over repetitive diving, compared to bounce diving. Therefore, a gradient reduction factor, η^{rep}, proportional to the difference between maximum and surface bubble inflation rate, is employed to maintain the separated phase volume below a limit point deduced from bounce and saturation diving data in the VPM and RGBM. Repetitive fractions are plotted for various tissue compartments (2, 10, 40, 120, 720 minutes) for surface intervals up to 200 minutes. Faster compartments are impacted the most, but all fractions relax to one after a few hours.

(2) ξ decrease with increasing exposure time;
(3) ξ increase with increasing surface interval time;
(4) ξ scale faster tissue compartments the most;
(5) ξ decrease with depth of dive segment;
(6) ξ scale deeper-than-previous dives the most;
(7) ξ is related to the regeneration time of micronuclei, τ_{reg}, the permissible bubble excess, Δn, and a time constant, τ_{rep}, characteristic of bubble inflation rate.

Consistent with the above set, Wienke constructed a multi-diving fraction from the micronuclei regeneration times, τ_{reg}, the excitation radii, r, and the characteristic time constant for permissible bubble excess in tissues, τ_{rep}. These ξ are written in product form, $\xi = \eta^{reg}\eta^{exc}\eta^{rep}$, with η^{reg} depending on micronuclei regeneration time, η^{exc} on excitation of additional nuclei on deeper-than-previous dives, and η^{rep} on bubble inflation rates on consecutive dives. All η are bounded by zero and one. Corresponding time scales

Figure 9b. Regeneration Factors.

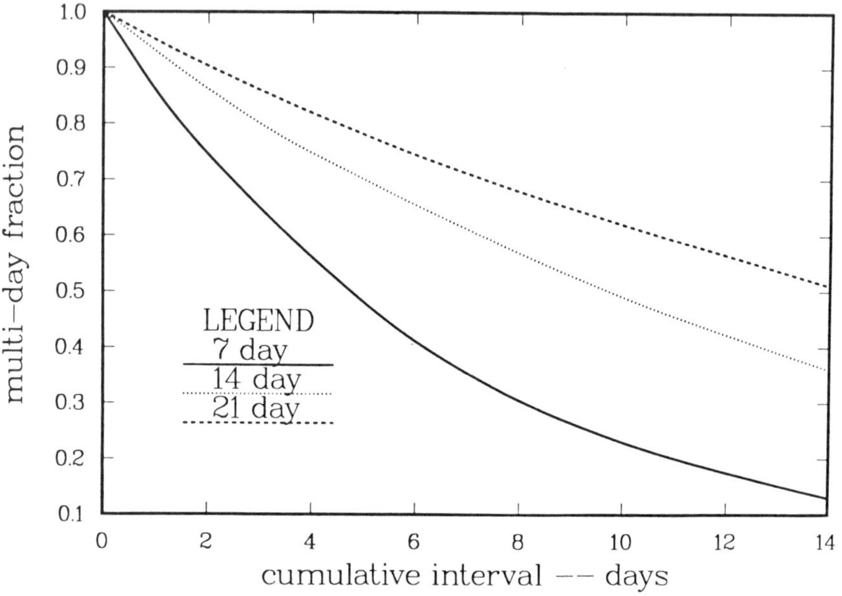

Micronuclei are thought to regenerate over adaptation time scales (days), contributing to existing pools of gas seeds. A factor, η^{reg}, accounting for creation of new micronuclei, reduces permissible gradients by the creation rate, thus maintaining the phase volume constraint over multi-day diving. Multi-day fractions are plotted for 7, 14, and 21 day regeneration times. Shorter regeneration times impart greater multi-day penalties.

for η are near $\tau_{reg} = 14$ *days*, and $\tau_{rep} = 40$ *minutes*. The (additional) excitation η^{exc} varies as the ratio of successive deeper-than-previous dive depths. Because elimination of free phases during surface intervals was not considered in the reduced gradient bubble model, the approach is conservative. Figures 9a, 9b, and 9c plot η^{rep}, η^{reg}, and η^{exc} for various cases, according to Appendix E.

In repetitive application, the multi-diving fractions, ξ, possess some general properties, consistent with the above checklist:

(1) reduce permissible bubble numbers, and hence repetitive bottom time;
(2) reduce permissible gradients, and hence multi-day exposures;
(3) penalize deeper-than-previous dives; and
(4) affect all tissue compartments, fast and slow.

Both τ_{reg} and τ_{rep} control repetitive diving, more particularly the critical parameters, *M* or *G*, with τ_{reg} mostly affecting multi-day and τ_{rep} mostly affecting repetitive activities. Six parameters, ξ, and *G* form the basis of the reduced gradient bubble model. Reduced non-stop time limits, restricted

Figure 9c. Excitation Factors.

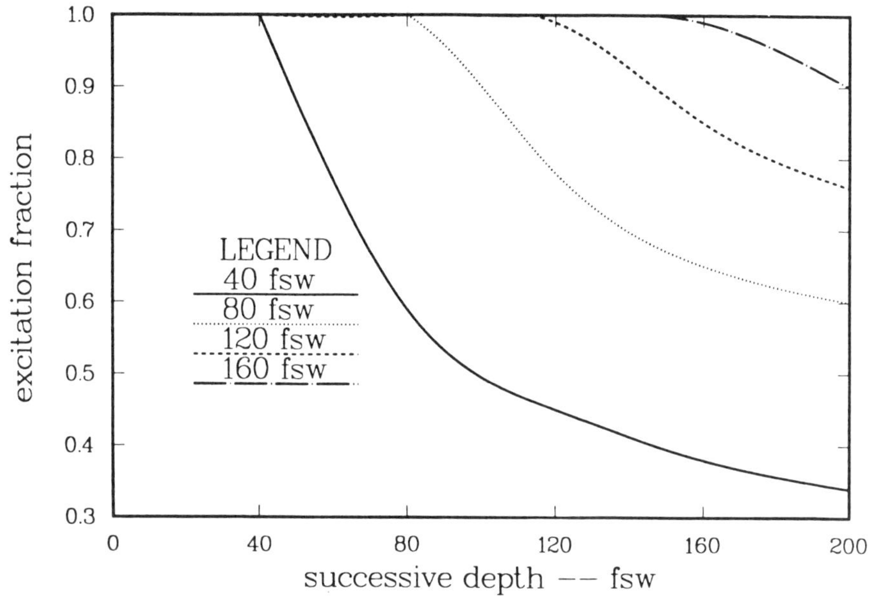

Deeper-than-previous diving activity stimulates smaller bubble seeds into growth according to the VPM and RGBM. Scaling gradients by the bubble excess on the present dive to the bubble excess on the deepest point of earlier dives, η^{exc}, also maintains the phase volume constraint for multi-exposures. Excitation fractions are plotted for a series of deeper exposures, following initial dives to 40, 80, 120, and 160 fsw. Shallow initial excursions, followed by deep dives, incur the largest reductions in permissible gradients on the deeper-than-previous dives.

deep repetitive diving, safety stops, deeper-than-previous dive limitations, and consistent treatment at altitude are all part of the algorithm, protocols consistent with bubbles, not only dissolved gas buildup.

As a simple demonstration of the model, consider two repetitive dives a day, 120 *fsw* for 10 *minutes* separated by a 2 *hr* surface interval, over three consecutive days. This profile, extended to three repetitive dives a day, has produced bends in 2 out of 3 cases on the first day, according to Leitch and Barnard, so it is not an academic exercise at this point. This bubble model reduces the permissible gradients in each tissue compartment, on each segment of the six dives, according to Table 6, listing ξ at the start of each repetitive and multi-day segment. Systematic reduction in ξ is clearly seen, correspondingly reducing non-stop exposure time. For application, each ξ in Table 6 multiplies the appropriate G from Table 5b.

Reductions in permissible gradients, and tensions to lesser degree, approach 20% in the fast compartments and 15% in the slower ones on the last dive. On the first day, reductions in the fast compartments approach 5%

Table 6. Multi-Diving Fractions (120 fsw/10 minutes, surface/120 minutes, twice a day for three days).

half-life τ *(minutes)*	fraction ξ_1	fraction ξ_2	fraction ξ_3	fraction ξ_4	fraction ξ_5	fraction ξ_6
1	1.00	.95	.93	.88	.86	.81
2	1.00	.95	.93	.88	.86	.81
5	1.00	.95	.93	.88	.86	.81
10	1.00	.95	.93	.89	.86	.82
20	1.00	.95	.93	.89	.86	.82
40	1.00	.96	.93	.89	.86	.82
80	1.00	.96	.93	.89	.86	.82
120	1.00	.96	.93	.90	.86	.82
180	1.00	.97	.93	.90	.86	.83
240	1.00	.97	.93	.90	.86	.84
360	1.00	.98	.93	.91	.86	.84
480	1.00	.98	.93	.91	.86	.85
720	1.00	1.00	.93	.93	.85	.85

on the second dive, and near 10% on the second dive of the second day. Smaller reductions, by a few percent, are seen in the slow compartments. Exposures in the 120 *fsw* range are controlled by the 10 *minute* compartment, with 11 *minutes* the non-stop time limit on the first dive ($\xi = 1$), from Table 6. On the sixth dive ($\xi = .82$), the non-stop limit drops to 6 *minutes* . On dives 2 through 5, non-stop time limits decrease monotonically between 11 and 7 *minutes.*

Such type bubble analyses are easily implemented in digital meters, with the inclusion of ξ, deduced from six model parameters, and G, extracted from a set of conservative non-stop limits, the essential components of the algorithm. Alternatively, the ξ can be freed from any model and extracted from exposure data. While there is relatively little multi-day and repetitive data now, testing programs such as those of Thalmann, Powell, and Rogers and the data gathering capabilities of hi-tech computers point to future possibilities.

CHAPTER 8

Mixed Gases

Nitrogen is limited as an inert gas for diving. Increased pressures of nitrogen beyond 200 *fsw* leads to excessive euphoria and reduced mental and physical functional ability, while beyond 600 *fsw* loss of consciousness results. Individual tolerances vary widely, often depending on activity. Symptoms can be marked at the beginning of a deep dive, gradually decreasing with time. Flow resistance and the onset of turbulence in the airways of the body increase with higher breathing gas pressure, considerably reducing ventilation with nitrogen-rich breathing mixtures during deep diving. Oxygen is also limited at depth for the usual toxicity reasons. Dives beyond 300 *fsw* requiring bottom times of hours need employ lighter, more weakly reacting, and less narcotic gases than nitrogen, and reduced oxygen partial pressures.

A number of inert gas replacements have been tested, such as hydrogen, neon, argon, and helium, with only helium and hydrogen performing satisfactorily on all counts. Because it is the lightest, hydrogen has elimination speed advantages over helium, but, because of the high explosive risk in mixing hydrogen, helium has emerged as the best all-round inert gas for deep and saturation diving. Helium can be breathed for months without tissue damage. Argon is highly soluble and heavier than nitrogen, and thus a very poor choice. Neon is not much lighter than nitrogen, but is only slightly more soluble than helium. Saturation and desaturation speeds of inert gases are inversely proprotional to the square root of their atomic masses. Hydrogen will saturate and desaturate approximately 3.7 times faster than nitrogen, and helium will saturate and desaturate some 2.7 times faster than nitrogen. Differences between neon, argon, and nitrogen are not significant for diving. Comparative properties of hydrogen, helium, neon, nitrogen, argon, and oxygen are listed in Table 7.

Table 7. Inert Gas And Oxygen Molecular Weights And Solubilities.

	H_2	*He*	*Ne*	N_2	*Ar*	O_2
A (amu)	**2.02**	**4.000**	**20.18**	**28.02**	**39.44**	**32.00**
S (ml/ml)						
blood	**.0149**	**.0087**	**.0093**	**.0122**	**.0260**	**.0241**
oil	**.0502**	**.0150**	**.0199**	**.0670**	**.1480**	**.1220**

The size of bubbles formed with various inert gases depends upon the amount of gas dissolved, and hence the solubilities. Higher gas solubilities promote bigger bubbles. Thus, helium is preferable to hydrogen as a light gas, while nitrogen is preferable to argon as a heavy gas. Neon solubility roughly equals nitrogen solubility.

Different uptake and elimination speeds suggest optimal means for reducing decompression time using helium and nitrogen mixtures. Following deep dives beyond 300 *fsw* breathing helium, switching to nitrogen is without risk, while helium elimination is accelerated because the helium tissue-blood gradient is increased when breathing an air mixture. By gradually increasing the oxygen content after substituting nitrogen for helium, the nitrogen uptake can also be kept low. Workable combinations of gas switching depend upon the exposure and the tissue compartment controlling the ascent. In deep saturation diving, *normoxic* breathing mixtures of gases are often advantageously employed to address oxygen concerns. A normoxic breathing mixture, helium or nitrogen, reduces the oxygen percentage so that the partial pressure of oxygen at the working depth is the same as at sea level.

Critical tensions can be employed in helium saturation diving in much the same fashion as nitrogen diving. A very simple approach to helium critical tensions in the slowest compartments employs the nitrogen tensions with the half-lives reduced by 2.7, that is, the helium half-lives are extracted from the nitrogen half-lives through division by 2.7, and the same critical tensions assumed for both half-lives. Tissue and critical tensions scale as the relative proportion of inert gas in the mixture. More so than in air diving, computational methods for mixed gas decompression and diving application are often proprietary information in the commercial sector. Helium (normal 80/20 mixture) non-stop time limits are shorter than nitrogen, as reported by Duffner, and follow a $dt_s^{1/2}$ law similar to nitrogen. Using the standard techniques of extracting critical tensions from the non-stop time limits, faster compartment critical tensions can be assigned for applications, as detailed by Workman. Bubbles models, such as the varying permeability model, have also been employed in helium saturation diving.

CHAPTER 9

Decompression Risk and Statistics

The systematics of gas exchange, nucleation, bubble growth and elimination, and decompression are so complicated that theories only reflect pieces of the puzzle. Computational algorithms, tables, and manned testing are requisite in a spectrum of diving activities. And the potential of electronic devices to process tables of information or detailed equations underwater is reaching maturity, with virtually any algorithm amenable to digital implementation. Pressures for even more sophisticated algorithms are expected to grow.

Still computational models enjoy varying degrees of success and failure, as discussed. More complex models address a greater number of issues, but are harder to codify in tables. The opposite is true for simpler models. Some models are based on first principles, but most are not. Application of models can be subjective in the absence of definitive data, the acquisition of which is tedious, sometimes controversial, and often ambiguous. When deterministic models are abandoned, statistical models can address the variability of outcome inherent to random occurrences, but only in grayer tones insofar as specification of controlling mechanisms. The dose-response characteristics of statistical models and data correlations are very attractive in the formulation of risk tables. Applied to decompression, tables of comparative statistical risk offer a means of weighing contributing factors and exposure alternatives.

9.1 PROBABILISTIC DECOMPRESSION

Biological processes are highly variable in outcome. Formal correlations with outcome statistics are then generally requisite to validate models. Often, this correlation is difficult to firmly (few percent) establish with fewer than a 1000 trial observations, while tens of percent correlations can be obtained with 30 trials, assuming binomial distributed probabilities. For decompression analysis, this works as a disadvantage, because often the trial space of dives is small. Not discounting the possibly small trial space, a probabilistic approach to the occurrence of decompression sickness is useful and necessary. One very successful approach, developed and tuned by Weathersby, Homer, Flynn, Hays, Survanshi, and others for decompression sickness in diving, called maximum likelihood, applies theory or models to diving data and adjusts the parameters until theoretical prediction and experimental data are in as close agreement as possible, as outlined in Appendix F.

Validation procedures require decisions about uncertainty. When a given decompression procedure is repeated with different subjects, or the same subjects on different occasions, the outcome is not constant. The uncertainty about the occurrence of decompression sickness can be quantified with statistical statements, though, suggesting limits to the validation procedure. For instance, after analyzing decompression incidence statistics for a set of procedures, a table designer may report that the procedure will offer an incidence rate below 5%, with 90% confidence in the statement. Alternatively, the table designer can compute the probability of rejecting a procedure using any number of dive trials, with the rejection criteria any arbitrary number of incidences. As the number of trials increases, the probability of rejecting a procedure increases for fixed incidence criteria. In this way, relatively simple statistical procedures can provide vital information as to the number of trials necessary to validate a procedure with any level of acceptable risk, or the maximum risk associated with any number of incidences and trials.

Decompression sickness is a hit, or (hopefully) no-hit situation. The statistics are binary, as in coin tossing. Probabilities of occurrence are determined by the binomial distribution. If we want to assign a probability to a hit, or no-hit situation, we can apply the binomial distribution (Appendix F) to the number of the dives, N, and the number of cases of decompression sickness, n. Table 8 lists the corresponding probability, for 1% and 10% underlying incidence, ρ, yielding 0, 1, and 2 or more cases of decompression sickness. The underlying incidence, ρ, is just the average number of hits. As the number of trials increases, the probability 0 or 1 incidences drops, while the probability of 2 or more incidences increases. In the case of 5 dives, the probability might be as low as 5%, while in the case of 50 dives, the probability could be 39%, both for $\rho = .01$. Clearly, odds even percentages would require testing beyond 50 cases for an underlying incidence near 1%. Only by increasing the number of trials for fixed incidences can the percentages be increased. Turning that around, a rejection procedure for 1 or more cases of decompression sickness at the 10% incidence level requires many more than 50 dives. If we are willing to lower the confidence of the acceptance, or rejection, procedure, of course, the number of requisite trials drops. Table 8 also shows that the standard test practice of accepting an exposure schedule following 10 trials without incidence of decompression sickness is suspect, merely because the relative probability of non-incidence is high, near 35%.

Table 8. Probability Of Decompression Sickness For 1% And 10% Underlying Incidence.

N(dives)	*n* (cases)	$\rho = .01$ $\sigma = .99$	$\rho = .10$ $\sigma = .90$
5	0	.95	.59
	1	.04	.33
	2 or more	.01	.08
10	0	.90	.35
	1	.09	.39
	2 or more	.01	.26
20	0	.82	.12
	1	.16	.27
	2 or more	.02	.61
50	0	.61	.01
	1	.31	.03
	2 or more	.08	.96

One constraint usually facing the statistical table designer is a paucity of data, that is, number of trials of a dive procedure. Data on hundreds of repetitions of a dive profile are virtually nonexistent, except bounce diving perhaps. As seen, some 30-50 trials are requisite to ascertain procedure safety at the 10% level. But 30-50 trials is probably asking too much, is too expensive, or generally prohibitive. In that case, the designer may try to employ global statistical measures linked to models in a more complex trial space, rather than a single profile trial space. Integrals of risk parameters, such as bubble number, supersaturation, separated phase, etc., over exposures in time, can be defined as probability measures for incidence of decompression sickness, and the maximum likelihood method then used to extract appropriate constants. Such an integrated approach using supersaturation risk was applied by Weathersby and co-workers to both air and helium tables.

9.2. RISK TABLES

The global statistical approach to the table fabrication consists of following a risk measure, or factor ρ, throughout and after sets of exposures, tallying the incidence of decompression, and then applying maximum likelihood to the risk integral in time, extracting any set of risk constants optimally over all dives in the maximization procedure. In analyzing recent data, risk was taken to be the difference between tissue tension and ambient pressure divided by ambient pressure. One tissue was assumed, with time constant ultimately fixed by the data in ensuing maximum likelihood analysis. The measure of incidence, ρ, was taken to be one minus the exponential of risk integrated over exposure time (Appendix F). Some 600 air dives were analyzed with this procedure, permitting construction of decompression schedules with 95% and 99% confidence (5% and 1% bends incidence). These tables have been published by Weathersby, Homer, Flynn, Survanshi, Hays, and colleagues.

Implicit in such formulations of risk tables are the assumptions that a given decompression stress is more likely to produce symptoms if it is sustained in time, and that large numbers of separate events may culminate in the same probability after time integration. Though individual schedule segments were not replicated enough to offer total statistical validation, categories of predicted safety were always found to be in accord with subsets of data. Since the method is general, any model parameter or meaningful index, properly normalized, can be applied to decompression data, and the full power of statistical methods employed to quantify overall risk. While powerful, such statistical methods are neither deterministic nor mechanistic, and cannot predict on first principles. But as a means to table fabrication with quoted risk, such approaches offer attractive pathways for analysis.

Validation procedures for schedules and tables can be quantified by a set of procedures based on statistical decompression analysis:

(1) select or construct a measure of decompression risk, or a probabilistic model;
(2) evaluate as many dives as possible, and especially those dives similar in exposure time, depth, and environmental factors;
(3) conduct limited testing if no data is available;
(4) apply the model to the data using maximum likelihood;
(5) construct appropriate schedules or tables using whatever incidence of decompression sickness is acceptable;
(6) release and then collect use statistics for final validation and tuning.

Questions of what risk is acceptable to the diver vary. Sport and research divers would probably opt for very small risk (1% or less), while military and commercial divers might live with higher risk (1-2%), considering the nearness of medical attention in general. Many factors influence these two populations, but fitness and acclimatization levels would probably differ considerably across them. While such factors are difficult to fold into any table exercise or analysis, the simple fact that human subjects in dive experiments exhibit higher incidences during testing phases certainly helps to lower the actual incidence rate in the field, noted by Bennett and Lanphier.

CHAPTER 10

Summary

Gas exchange, bubble formation and elimination, and compression-decompression in blood and tissues are governed by many factors, such as diffusion, perfusion, phase separation and equilibration, nucleation and cavitation, local fluid shifts, and combinations thereof. Owing to the complexity of biological systems, multiplicity of tissues and media, diversity of interfaces and boundary conditions, and plethora of bubble impacting physical and chemical mechanisms, it is difficult to solve the decompresssion problem *in vivo*. Early decompression studies adopted the supersaturation viewpoint. Closer looks at the physics of phase separation and bubbles in the mid-1970s, and insights into gas transfer mechanisms, culminated in extended kinetics and dissolved-free phase theories. Integration of both approaches can proceed on the numerical side because calculational techniques can be made equivalent. Phase and bubble models are more general than supersaturation models, incorporating their predictive capabilities as subsets. Statistical models, developed mostly in the mid-1980s, are gray from mechanistic viewpoint, but offer the strongest correlations with actual experiments and exposures, possibly the best approach to table fabrication.

Computation models gain efficacy by their ability to track data, often independent from physical interpretation. In that sense, the bottom line for computational models is utility, operational reliability, and reproducibility. Correct models can achieve such ends, but almost any model with sufficient parameter latitude could achieve those same ends. It is fair to say that deterministic models admit varying degrees of computational license, that model parameters may not correlate as complete set with the real world, and that not all mechanisms are addressed optimally. That is, perhaps, one reason why we see representative diving sectors, such as sport, military, commercial, and research, employing different tables, meters, models, and algorithms. Yet, given this situation, phase models attempting to treat both free and dissolved gas exchange, bubbles and gas nuclei, and free phase trigger points appear preferable to less comprehensive models. Phase models have the right physical signatures, and thus the potential to extrapolate reasonably when confronting new applications and data.

References

(1) Abramowitz M. and Stegun I.A., 1972, *"Handbook Of Mathematical Functions",* New York: Dover Publications.

(2) Albano G., Griscuoli P.M., and Ciulla C., 1962, "La Sindrome Neuropsichica Di Profundita", *Lav. Um.* 14, 351-358.

(3) Atkins C.E., Lehner C.E., Beck K.A., Dubielzig R.R., Nordheim E.V., and Lanphier E.H., 1988, "Experimental Respiratory Decompression Sickness in Sheep", *J. Appl. Physiol.* 65, 1163-1171.

(4) Bassett B.E., 1979, "And Yet Another Approach To The Problems Of Altitude Diving And Flying After Diving", *Decompression In Depth Proceedings,* Professional Association of Diving Instructors, Santa Ana.

(5) Bateman J.B. and Lang J., 1945, "Formation And Growth of Bubbles In Aqueous Solutions", *Canad. J. Res.* E23, 22-31.

(6) Behnke A.R., 1967, "The Isobaric (Oxygen Window) Principle Of Decompression", *Trans. Third Annual Conf. Marine Tech, Soc.* 1, 213-228.

(7) Behnke A.R., 1937, "The Application Of Measurements of Nitrogen Elimination To The Problem Of Decompressing Divers", *USN Med. Bull.* 35, 219-240.

(8) Bell R.L. and Borgwardt R.E., 1976, "The Theory Of High Altitude Correction To The U.S. Navy Standard Decompression Tables: I. The Cross Corrections", *Undersea Biomed. Res.* 3, 1-23.

(9) Bennett P.B. and Elliot D.H., 1969, "The Physiology And Medicine Of Diving And Compressed Air Work", London: Bailliere Tindall And Cassell.

(10) Berghage T.E., Armstrong F.W., and Conda K.J., 1975, "Relationship Between Saturation Exposure Pressure And Subsequent Decompression In Mice", *Aviat. Space Environ. Med.* 46, 224-247.

(11) Bert P., 1878, "La Pression Barometrique", Paris: Masson.

(12) Boni M., Schibli R., Nussberger P., and Buhlmann A.A., 1976, "Diving At Diminished Atmospheric Pressure: Air Decompression Tables For Different Altitudes", *Undersea Biomed. Res.* 3, 189-204.
(13) Bowker A.H. and Lieberman G.J., 1964, "Engineering Statistics", Englewood Cliffs: Prentice-Hall Inc.
(14) Boycott A.E., Damant G.C.C., and Haldane J.S., 1908, "The Prevention Of Compressed-Air Illness", *J. Hyg.* 8, 342-443.
(15) Buckles R.G., 1968, "The Physics Of Bubble Formation And Growth", *Aerospace Med.* 39, 1062-1069.
(16) Buhlmann A.A., 1984, "Decompression/Decompression Sickness", Berlin: Springer-Verlag.
(17) Carslaw H.S. and Jaeger J.C., 1950, "Conduction Of Heat In Solids", Oxford: Clarendon Press.
(18) Crocker W.E., Goodenough F.C., and Davidson W.M., 1951, "Investigation Into The Decompression Tables: Progress Report On The First Series Of Human Exposures", *Medical Research Council Report,* UPS 118, London.
(19) Crocker W.E. and Taylor H.J., 1952, "A Method Of Calculating Decompression Stages And The Formulation Of New Diving Tables", *Investigation Into The Decompression Tables, Medical Research Council Report,* UPS 131, London.
(20) Cross E.R., 1970, "High Altitude Decompression", *Skin Diver Magazine* 19, 17-18.
(21) Davidson W.M., Sutton B.M., and Taylor H.J., 1950, "Decompression Ratio For Goats Following Long Exposure And Return To Atmospheric Pressure Without Stoppage", *Medical Research Council Report,* UPS 110, London.
(22) Des Granges M., 1957, "Repetitive Diving Decompression Tables", *US Navy Experimental Diving Unit Report,* NEDU 6-57, Washington, D.C.
(23) Duffner G.J., Synder J.F., and Smith L.L., 1959, "Adaptation Of Helium-Oxygen To Mixed Gas Scuba", *US Navy Experimental Diving Unit Report,* NEDU 3-59, Washington, D.C.
(24) Dwyer J.V., 1956, "Calculation Of Repetitive Diving Decompression Tables", *US Navy Experimental Diving Unit Report,* NEDU 1-57, Washington, D.C.
(25) Edel P.O., Carroll J.J., Honaker R.W., and Beckman E.L., 1969, "Interval At Sea-Level Pressure Required To Prevent Decompression Sickness In Humans Who Fly In Commercial Aircraft After Diving", *Aerospace Med.* 40, 1105-1110.
(26) Epstein P.S. and Plesset M.S., 1950, "On The Stability Of Gas Bubbles In Liquid-Gas Solutions", *J. Chm. Phys.* 18, 1505-1509.
(27) Evans A. and Walder D.N., 1969, "Significance Of Gas Macronuclei In The Aetiology Of Decompression Sickness", *Nature London* 222, 251-252.

(28) Farm F.P., Hayashi E.M., and Beckman E.L., 1986, "Diving And Decompression Sickness Treatment Practices Among Hawaii's Diving Fisherman", *University of Hawaii Sea Grant Report,* UNIHI-SEA-GRANT-TP-86-01, Honolulu.

(29) Fulton J.F., 1951, *"Decompression Sickness"*, Philadelphia: Saunders Publishing Co.

(30) Gernhardt M.L., 1985, "Tissue Gas Bubble Dynamics During Hypobaric Exposures", *Society Of Automotive Engineers Report,* SAE-851337, Warrendale.

(31) Gernhardt M.L., Lambertsen C.J., Miller R.G., and Hopkins E., 1990, "Evaluation Of A Theoretical Model Of Tissue Gas Phase Growth And Resolution During Decompression From Air Diving", *Undersea Biomed. Res.* 17, 95.

(32) Golding F.C., Griffiths P.D., Paton W.D.M., Walder D.N., and Hempleman H.V., 1960, "Decompression Sickness During Construction Of The Dartford Tunnel", *Brit. J. Ind. Med.* 17, 167-180.

(33) Gray J.S., Masland R.L., and Mahady S.C., 1945, "The Effects Of Breathing Carbon Dioxide On Altitude Decompression Sickness", *US Air Force School of Aviation Medicine Report,* Project 409, Randolph Field.

(34) Hamilton R.W., 1975, "Development Of Decompression Procedures For Depths In Excess Of 400 Feet", *Undersea And Hyperbaric Medical Society Report,* WS: 2-28-76, Bethesda.

(35) Harvey E.N., 1945, "Decompression Sickness And Bubble Formation In Blood And Tissue", *Bull. N.Y. Acad. Med.* 21, 505-536.

(36) Harvey E.N., Barnes D.K., McElroy W.D., Whiteley A.H., Pease D.C., and Cooper K.W., 1944, "Bubble Formation In Animals. I. Physical Factors", *J. Cell Comp. Physiol.* 24, 1-22.

(37) Harvey E.N., McElroy W.D., Whiteley A.H., Warren G.H., and Pease D.C., 1944, "Bubble Formation In Animals. III. An Analysis Of Gas Tension And Hydrostatic Pressure in Cats", *J. Cell Comp. Physiol.* 24, 117-132.

(38) Harvey E.N., Whiteley A.H., McElroy W.D., Pease D.C., and Barnes D.K., 1944, "Bubble Formation In Animals. II. Gas Nuclei And Their Distribution In Blood And Tissues", *J. Cell Comp. Physiol.* 24, 23-24.

(39) Hawkins J.A., Shilling C.W., and Hansen R.A., 1935, "A Suggested Change In Calculating Decompression Tables For Diving", *USN Med. Bull.* 33, 327-338.

(40) Hempleman H.V., 1957, "Further Basic Facts On Decompression Sickness", *Investigation Into The Decompression Tables, Medical Research Council Report,* UPS 168, London.

(41) Hempleman H.V., 1952, "A New Theoretical Basis For The Calculation Of Decompression Tables", *Investigation Into The Decompression Tables, Medical Research Council Report,* UPS 131, London.

(42) Hennessy T.R. 1974, "The Interaction Of Diffusion And Perfusion In Homogenous Tissue", *Bull. Math. Biol.* 36, 505-527.
(43) Hennessy T.R. and Hempleman H.V., 1977, "An Examination Of The Critical Released Gas Concept In Decompression Sickness", *Proc. Royal Soc. London* B197, 299-313.
(44) Hill A.V., 1928, "Diffusion of O_2 And Lactic Acid Through Tissues", *Proc. Royal Soc.* B104, 39-96.
(45) Hills B.A., 1977, *"Decompression Sickness",* New York: John Wiley And Sons Inc.
(46) Hills B.A., 1969, "Radial Bulk Diffusion Into Heterogeneous Tissue", *Bull Math. Biophysics* 31, 25-34.
(47) Hills B.A., 1968 "Linear Bulk Diffusion Into Heterogeneous Tissue", *Bull. Math. Biophysics* 30, 47-59.
(48) Hills B.A., 1968, "Relevant Phase Conditions For Predicting The Occurrence Of Decompression Sickness", *J. Appl. Physiol.* 25, 310-315.
(49) Hills B.A., 1968, "Variation In Susceptibility To Decompression Sickness", *Int. J. Biometeor.* 12, 343-349.
(50) Hills B.A., 1967; "Decompression Sickness: A Study Of Cavitation At The Liquid-Liquid Interface", *Aerospace Med.* 38, 814-817.
(51) Hills B.A., 1967, "Diffusion Versus Blood Perfusion In Limiting The Rate Of Uptake Of Inert Non-Polar Gases By Skeletal Rabbit Muscle", *Clin. Sci.* 33, 67-87.
(52) Huggins K.E., 1987, "Multiprocessor Applications To Multi-Level Air Decompression Problems", *Michigan Sea Grant Publication,* MICHU-SG-87-201, Ann Arbor.
(53) Inman V.T. and Saunders J.B., 1944, "Referred Pain From Skeletal Structures", *Mental Dis.* 99, 660-667.
(54) Irving J. and Mullineux N., 1972, "Mathematics In Physics And Engineering", London: Academic Press Inc.
(55) Keller H. and Buhlmann A.A., 1965, "Deep Diving And Short Decompression By Breathing Mixed Gases", *J. Appl. Physiol.* 20, 1267.
(56) Kety S.S., 1951, "The Theory And Applications Of The Exchange Of Inert Gases At The Lungs And Tissues", *Pharm. Rev.* 3, 1-41.
(57) Kety S.S. and Schmidt C.F., 1945, "The Determination Of Cerebral Blood Flow In Man By Use Of Nitrous Oxide In Low Concentrations", *Amer. J. Physiol.* 143, 53-56.
(58) Krogh A., 1918, "The Rate Of Invasion Of Gases Through Animal Tissue, With Some Remarks On The Coefficient Of Invasion", *J. Physiol.* 52, 391.
(59) Kunkle T.D. and Beckman E.L., 1983, "Bubble Dissolution Physics And The Treatment Of Decompression Sickness", *Med. Phys.* 10, 184-190.

(60) Lang M.A. and Egstrom G.H., 1990, "Proceedings Of The American Academy Of Underwater Sciences Biomechanics Of Safe Ascents Workshop", *American Academy Of Underwater Sciences Diving Safety Publication,* AAUSDSP-BSA-01-90, Costa Mesa.

(61) Lang M.A. and Hamilton R.W., 1989, *"Proceedings Of The American Academy Of Underwater Sciences Dive Computer Workshop",* University Of Southern California Sea Grant Publication, USCSG-TR-01-89, Los Angeles.

(62) Lanphier E.H. and Lehner C.E., 1982, "An Unrecognized Hazard Of Altitude", *Pressure* 11,4.

(63) Lehner C.E., Hei D.J., Palta M., Lightfoot E.N., and Lanphier E.H., 1988, "Accelerated Onset Of Decompression Sickness In Sheep After Short Deep Dives," *University Of Wisconsin Sea Grant College Program Report,* WIS-SG-88-843, Madison.

(64) Leitch D.R. and Barnard E.E.P., 1982, "Observations On No-Stop And Repetitive Air And Oxynitrogen Diving", *Undersea Biomed. Res.* 9, 113-129.

(65) LeMessurier D.H. and Hills B.A., 1965, "Decompression Sickness: A Study Of Diving Techniques In The Torres Strait", *Hvaldradets Skrifter* 48, 54-84.

(66) Mathews J. and Walker R.L., 1975, Mathematical Methods of Physics", New York: W.A. Benjamin Inc.

(67) Nishi R.Y., 1978, "Real-Time Decompression Monitoring By Computers", *Defense and Civil Institute Of Environmental Medicine Report,* DCIEM 78-X-27, Ontario.

(68) Paton W.D.M. and Walder D.N., 1954, "Compressed Air Illness", *Medical Research Council Report,* HMSO 281, London.

(69) Pilmanis A.A., 1976, "Intravenous Gas Emboli In Man after Compressed Air Ocean Diving", Office Of Naval Research Contract Report, N00014-67-A-0269-0026, Washington, D.C.

(70) Powell C.F., 1928, "Condensation Phenomena At Different Temperatures", *Proc. Royal Soc. London* A119, 553-577.

(71) Powell R.P. and Rogers R.E., 1989, "Doppler Ultrasound Monitoring Of Gas Phase Formation And Resolution In Repetitive Diving", *Undersea Biomed. Res.* 16, 69.

(72) Rashbass C., 1955, "New Tables", *Investigation Into The Decompression Tables, Medical Research Council Report,* UPS 151, London.

(73) Rogers R.E. and Powell M.R., 1989, "Controlled Hyperbaric Chamber Tests Of Multi-Day Repetitive Dives", *Undersea Biomed. Res.* 16, 68.

(74) Roughton F.J.W., 1952, "Diffusion And Chemical Reaction Velocity In Cylindrical And Spherical Systems Of Physiological Interest", *Proc. Royal Soc.* B140, 203-221.

(75) Sagan H., 1971, "Boundary And Eigenvalue Problems In Mathematical Physics", New York: John Wiley And Sons Inc.

(76) Schreiner H.R. and Hamilton R.W., 1987, "Validation Of Decompression Tables", *Undersea And Hyperbaric Medical Society Publication 74* (VAL), Bethesda.

(77) Sheffield P.J., 1990, "Flying After Diving", *Undersea And Hyperbaric Medical Society Publication 77* (FLYDIV), Bethesda.

(78) Smith C.L., 1975, "Altitude Procedures For The Ocean Diver", *National Association of Underwater Instructors Technical Publication 5,* Colton.

(79) Spencer M.P., 1976 "Decompression Limits For Compressed Air Determined By Ultrasonically Detected Blood Bubbles", *J. Appl. Physiol.* 40, 229-235.

(80) Spencer M.P., and Campbell S.D., 1968, "The Development Of Bubbles In The Venous And Arterial Blood During Hyperbaric Decompression", *Bull. Mason Cli.* 22, 26-32.

(81) Strauss R.H., 1974, "Bubble Formation In Gelatin: Implications For Prevention Of Decompression Sickness", *Undersea Biomed. Res.* 1, 169-174.

(82) Tepper R.S., Lightfoot E.N., Baz A., and Lanphier E.H. 1979, "Inert Gas Transport In The Microcirculation: Risk Of Isobaric Supersaturation", *J. Apply Physiol.* 46, 1157-1163.

(83) Thalmann E.D., 1986, "Air-N_2O_2 Decompression Computer Development", *US Navy Experimental Diving Unit Report,* NEDU 8-85, Panama City.

(84) Thalmann E.D., 1984, "Phase II Testing Of Decompression Algorithms For Use In The US Navy Underwater Decompression Computer", *US Navy Experimental Diving Unit Report,* NEDU 1-84, Panama City.

(85) Thalman E.D. and Spaur W.H., 1980, "Testing Of Decompression Algorithms For Use In The US Navy Underwater Decompression Computer", *US Navy Experimental Diving Unit Report,* NEDU 11-80, Groton.

(86) Thompson A.M., Cavert H.M., and Lifson N., 1958, "Kinetics Of D_2O And Antipyrine In Isolated Perfused Rat Liver", *Amer. J. Physiol.* 192, 531-537.

(87) Van Liew H.D., Bishop B., Walder P.D., and Rahn H., 1975, "Bubble Growth And Mechanical Properties Of Tissue In Decompression", *Undersea Biomed. Res.* 2, 185-194.

(88) Vann R.D. and Clark H.G., 1975, "Bubble Growth And Mechanical Properties Of Tissue In Decompression", *Undersea Biomed. Res.* 2, 185-194.

(89) Vann R.D., Dovenbarger J., Wachholz C., and Bennett P.B., 1989, "Decompression Sickness In Dive Computer And Table Use", *DAN Newsletter* 3-6.

(90) Walder D.N., 1968, "Adaptation To Decompression Sickness In Caisson Work", *Biometeor.* 11, 350-359.

(91) Walder D.N., Evans A., and Hempleman H.V., 1968, "Ultrasonic Monitoring Of Decompression", *Lancet.* 1, 897-898.
(92) Weathersby P.K., Homer L.D., and Flynn E.T., 1984, "On The Likelihood Of Decompression Sickness", *J. Appl. Physiol.* 57, 815-825.
(93) Weathersby P.K., Survanshi S., and Homer L.D., 1985, "Statistically Based Decompression Tables. I. Analysis Of Standard Air Dives: 1950-1970", *Naval Medical Research Institute Report,* NMRI 85-16, Bethesda.
(94) Weathersby P.K., Survanshi S., and Homer L.D., 1985, "Statistically Based Decompression Tables. II. Equal Risk Air Decompression Tables", *Naval Medical Research Institute Report,* NMRI 85-17, Bethesda.
(95) Wienke B.R., 1991, "High Altitude Diving", *National Association of Underwater Instructors Technical Publication,* Montclair.
(96) Wienke B.R., 1990, "Reduced Gradient Bubble Model", *Int. J. Bio-Med. Comp.* 26, 232-256.
(97) Wienke B.R., 1990, "Modeling Dissolved And Free Phase Gas Dynamics Under Decompression", *Int. J. Bio-Med. Comp.* 25, 193-205.
(98) Wienke B.R., 1989, "Equivalent Multi-Tissue And Thermodynamic Decompression Algorithms", *Int. J. Bio-Med. Comp.* 24, 227-245.
(99) Wienke B.R., 1989, "N_2 Transfer And Critical Pressure In Tissue Compartments", *Math. Comp. Model.* 12, 1-15.
(100) Wienke B.R., 1989, "Tissue Gas Exchange Models And Decompression Computations: A Review", *Undersea Biomed. Res.* 16, 53-89.
(101) Wienke B.R., 1987, "Computational Decompression Models", *Int. J. Bio-Med. Comp.* 21, 205-221.
(102) Wienke B.R., 1986, "DECOMP: Computational Package For Nitrogen Transport Modeling In Tissues", *Comp. Phys. Comm.* 40, 327-336.
(103) Wienke B.R., 1986, "Phenomenological Models For Nitrogen Transport In Tissues", *Il Nuovo Cimento* 8D, 417-435.
(104) Wienke B.R and Graver D.K., 1991, "Multi-Level Decompression Table Procedure Revisited", *Sources* (in press).
(105) Wienke B.R and Hills B.A., 1989, *"Bubbles And Bends And Bio-transport",* New York: Marcel Dekker Inc.
(106) Wittenborn A.F., 1963, "An Analytic Development Of A Decompression Computer", *Proc. Second Symp. Underwater Physiol.,* Washington D.C.: National Academy Of Science 1, 82-90.
(107) Workman R.D., 1965, "Calculation Of Decompression Schedules for Nitrogen-Oxygen And Helium-Oxygen Dives", *US Navy Experimental Diving Unit Report,* NEDU 6-65, Washington, D.C.
(108) Yarborough O.D., 1937, "Calculations Of Decompression Tables", *US Navy Experimental Diving Unit Research Report,* Washington, D.C.
(109) Yount D.E., 1982, "On The Evolution, Generation, And Regeneration Of Gas Cavitation Nuclei", *J. Acoust. Soc. Am.* 71, 1473-1481.

(110) Yount D.E., 1979, "Skins Of Varying Permeability: A Stabilization Mechanism For Gas Cavitation Nuclei", *J. Acoust. Soc. Am.* 65, 1431-1439.
(111) Yount D.E., Gillary E.W., and Hoffman D.C., 1984, "A Microscopic Investigation Of Bubble Formation Nuclei", *J. Acoust. Soc. Am.* 76, 1511-1521.
(112) Yount D.E. and Hoffman D.C., 1986 "On The Use Of A Bubble Formation Model To Calculate Diving Tables", *Aviat. Space Environ. Med.* 57, 149-156.
(113) Yount D.E. and Strauss R.H., 1976, "Bubble Formation In Gelatin: A Model For Decompression Sickness", *J. Appl. Phys.* 47, 5081-5089.
(114) Yount D.E., Yeung C.M., and Ingle F.W., 1979, "Determination Of The Radii Of Gas Cavitation Nuclei by Filtering Gelatin", *J. Acoust. Soc. Am.* 65, 1440-1450.

Appendices

The Appendices detail mathematical aspects mentioned, but not developed, in the text. They include tissue gas exchange, critical tensions and volumes, nucleation and bubbles, and decompression risk. They are appended for completeness, and directed toward the more interested reader.

APPENDIX A: PERFUSION LIMITED EXCHANGE

Exchange of inert gas, controlled by blood flow rates across regions of varying concentration, is driven by the local gradient, that is, the difference between the arterial blood tension, p_a, and the instantaneous tissue tension p. Such behavior is modeled in time, t, by simple classes of exponential response functions, bounded by p_a and the initial value of p, denoted p_i. These multi-tissue functions satisfy a differential perfusion rate equation,

$$\frac{\partial p}{\partial t} = -\lambda\,(p - p_a), \qquad \text{(A-1)}$$

and take the form, tracking both dissolved gas buildup and elimination symmetrically,

$$p - p_a = (p_i - p_a)\,exp\,(-\lambda t),$$

$$\lambda = \frac{.6931}{\tau}, \qquad \text{(A-2)}$$

with perfusion constant, λ, defined by the tissue half-time, τ. Compartments with 1, 2.5, 5, 10, 20, 40, 80, 120, 180, 240, 360, 480, and 720 minute half-lives, τ, are employed, and half-lives are independent of pressure.

In a series of dives or multiple stages, p_i and p_a represent extremes for each stage, or more precisely, the initial tension and the arterial tension at the beginning of the next stage. Stages are treated sequentially, with finishing tensions at one step representing initial tensions for the next step, and so on. To maximize the rate of uptake or elimination of dissolved gases the *gradient,* simply the difference between p_i and p_a, is maximized by pulling the diver as close to the surface as possible. Exposures are limited by requiring that the tissue tensions never exceed M, written,

$$M = M_0 + \Delta M\, d, \tag{A-3}$$

as a function of depth, d, for ΔM the change per unit depth. A set of M_0 and ΔM are listed in Table 1. In absolute units, the corresponding critical gradient, G, is given by,

$$G = \frac{M}{.79} - P, \tag{A-4}$$

with P ambient pressure, and M critical nitrogen pressure.

At altitude, some critical tensions have been correlated with actual testing, in which case, the depth, d, is defined in terms of the absolute pressure,

$$d = P - 33, \tag{A-5}$$

with surface pressure, P_0, at altitude, z, given by *(fsw),*

$$P_0 = 33\, exp\,(-0.0381\, z) = 33\, \alpha^{-1},$$

$$\alpha = exp\,(0.0381\, z), \tag{A-6}$$

and z in multiples of 1000 *feet*. However, in those cases where the critical tensions have not been tested nor extended to altitude, an exponentially decreasing extrapolation scheme, called *similarity,* has been employed. Extrapolations of critical tensions, below $P = 33$ *fsw*, then fall off more rapidly than in the linear case, Eq. (A-5). The similarity extrapolation holds the ratio, $R = M/P$, constant at altitude. Denoting an equivalent sea level depth, δ, at altitude, z, one has for an excursion to depth d,

$$\frac{M(d)}{d + 33\alpha^{-1}} = \frac{M(\delta)}{\delta + 33}, \tag{A-7}$$

so that the equality is satisfied when,

$$\delta = \alpha d$$

$$M(\delta) = \alpha M(\mathrm{d}) \qquad \text{(A-8)}$$

Considering the minimum surface tension pressure of bubbles, G^{min} (near 10 *fsw*), as a limit point, the similarity extrapolation should be limited to 10000 *feet* in elevation, and neither for decompression, nor heavy repetitive diving.

As described in Appendix B, depth-time exposures are often limited by a law of the form,

$$d\, t_s^{1/2} = H\,, \qquad \text{(A-9)}$$

with t_s the non-stop time limit, and $400 \leq H \leq 500$ *fsw* $\mathrm{min}^{1/2}$. One can obtain the corresponding tissue constant, λ, controlling the exposure at depth d, for non-stop time t_s, by differentiating Eq. (A-2) with respect to depth, d, and setting the result to zero. With $p_a = .79\,(d + 33)$ at sea level, there results,

$$1 - exp\,(-\lambda t_s)(1 + 2\lambda t_s) = 0. \qquad \text{(A-10)}$$

Corresponding critical tensions, M, are then easily obtained from Eq. (A-2) using d, λ, and t_s. In the above case, the transcendental equation is satisfied when,

$$\lambda t_s = 1.25 \qquad \text{(A-11)}$$

Time remaining before a stop, time at a stop, or surface interval before flying can all be obtained by inverting Eq. (A-2). Denoting the appropriate critical tension at some desired stage, M, and the instantaneous tension at that time, p, at stage, p_a, the time remaining, t_{rem}, follows from,

$$t_{rem} = \frac{1}{\lambda}\, ln \left[\frac{p - p_a}{M - p_a} \right], \qquad \text{(A-12)}$$

for each compartment, λ. Obviously, the smallest t_{rem} controls the ascent.

APPENDIX B: DIFFUSION LIMITED EXCHANGE

Exchange of inert gas, controlled by diffusion across regions of varying concentration, is also driven by the local gradient. As before, denoting the arterial blood tension, p_a, and instantaneous tissue tension, p, the gas diffusion equation takes the form in one-dimensional planar geometry,

$$D \frac{\partial^2 p}{\partial x^2} = \frac{\partial p}{\partial t}, \quad \text{(B-1)}$$

with D a single diffusion coefficient appropriate to the media. Using standard techniques of separation of variables, with ω^2 the separation constant (eigenvalue), the solution is written,

$$p - p_a = (p_i - p_a) \sum_{n=1}^{\infty} W_n \sin(\omega_n x) \exp(-\omega_n^2 Dt), \quad \text{(B-2)}$$

assuming at the left tissue boundary, $x = 0$, we have $p = p_a$, and with W_n a set of constants obtained from the initial condition. First, requiring $p = p_a$ at the right tissue boundary, $x = l$, yields,

$$\omega_n = \frac{n\pi}{b}, \quad \text{(B-3)}$$

for all n. Then, taking $p = p_i$ at $t = 0$, multiplying both sides of Eq. (B-2) by $\sin(\omega_m x)$, integrating over the tissue zone, l, and collecting terms gives,

$$W_{2n} = 0,$$

$$W_{2n-1} = \frac{4}{(2n - 1)\pi}, \quad \text{(B-4)}$$

Averaging the solution over the tissue domain eliminates spatial dependence, that is $\sin(\omega_n x)$, from the solution, yields a bulk response,

$$p - p_a = (p_i - p_a) \sum_{n=1}^{\infty} \frac{8}{(2n - 1)^2 \pi^2} \exp(-\omega_{2n-1}^2 Dt). \quad \text{(B-5)}$$

The expansion resembles a weighted sum over *effective* tissue compartments with time constants, $\omega^2_{2n-1} D$, determined by diffusivity and boundary conditions.

Diffusion models fit the time constant, K,

$$K = \frac{\pi^2 D}{l^2}, \quad \text{(B-6)}$$

to exposure data, with a typical value employed by the Royal Navy given by,

$$K = 0.007928 \ \text{min}^{-1}. \tag{B-7}$$

The approach is aptly single tissue, with equivalent tissue half-life, τ_D,

$$\tau_D = \frac{.6931}{K} = 87.5 \ \textit{minutes}, \tag{B-8}$$

close to the US Navy 120 *minute* compartment used to control saturation, decompression, and repetitive diving. Corresponding critical tensions in the bulk model, take the form,

$$M = \frac{709\,P}{P + 404}, \tag{B-9}$$

falling somewhere between fixed gradient and multi-tissue values. At the surface, $M = 53$ *fsw,* while at 200 *fsw,* $M = 259$ *fsw.* A critical gradient, G satisfies,

$$G = \frac{M}{.79} - P = \frac{P\,(493 - P)}{(P + 404)}. \tag{B-10}$$

The limiting features of bulk diffusion can be gleaned from an extension of the above slab model in the limit of thick tissue region, that is, $l \longrightarrow \infty$. Replacing the summation over n in Eq. (B-5) with an integral as $l \longrightarrow \infty$, we find

$$p - p_a = (p_i - p_a)\ \overline{erf}\,[l/(4Dt)^{1/2}], \tag{B-11}$$

with $\overline{erf}$ the average value of the *error-function* over l having the limiting form, according to Abramowitz and Stegun,

$$\overline{erf}\,[l/(4Dt)^{1/2}] \approx 1 - \frac{(4Dt)^{1/2}}{l\pi^{1/2}}, \tag{B-12}$$

for short times, and

$$\overline{erf}\,[l/(4Dt)^{1/2}] \approx \frac{l}{(4\pi Dt)^{1/2}}, \tag{B-13}$$

for long times.

Unlike Eq. (A-2), the diffusion Eq. (B-2), consisting of a sum of exponentials in time, cannot be formally inverted to yield time remaining, time at a stop, nor time before flying. Such information can only be obtained by solving Eq. (B-2) numerically, that is, with computer or hand calculator for given M, p, and p_a.

If we wrap the above planar geometry around into a hollow cylinder of inner radius, a, and outer radius, b, we generate Krogh geometry. The hollow cylindrical model retains all the features of the planar model, and additionally includes curvature for small a and b, with $1 = b - a$ from before. Assigning the same boundary conditions at a and b, namely that the tissue tension, p, equals the arterial tension, p_a, writing the diffusion equation in radial cylindrical coordinates,

$$D \frac{\partial^2 p}{\partial r^2} + \frac{D}{r} \frac{\partial p}{\partial r} = \frac{\partial p}{\partial t} , \tag{B-14}$$

and solving yields,

$$p - p_a = (p_i - p_a) \sum_{n=1}^{\infty} X_n \, U_0(\epsilon_n r) \exp(-\epsilon_n^2 Dt) , \tag{B-15}$$

with X_n a constant satisfying initial conditions, U_0 the cylinder functions (see Abramowitz and Stegun), and ϵ_n the eigenvalues satisfying,

$$U_0(\epsilon_n a) = \frac{\partial U_0(\epsilon_n b/2)}{\partial r} = 0 . \tag{B-16}$$

Averaging over the tissue region, $a \leq r \leq b$, finally gives,

$$p - p_a = (p_i - p_a) \frac{4}{(b/2)^2 - a^2} \sum_{n=1}^{\infty} \frac{1}{\epsilon_n^2} \frac{J_1^2(\epsilon_n b/2)}{J_0^2(\epsilon_n a) - J_1^2(\epsilon_n b/2)} \exp(-\epsilon_n^2 Dt) , \tag{B-17}$$

with J_1 and J_0 Bessel functions, order 1 and 0. Typical vascular parameters are bounded roughly by,

$$0 < a \leq 4 \textit{ microns} ,$$

$$10 \leq b \leq 32 \textit{ microns} .$$

APPENDIX C: THERMODYNAMIC MODEL

The thermodynamic model couples both the tissue diffusion and blood perfusion equations. Cylindrical symmetry is assumed in the model. From a boundary vascular zone of thickness, *a,* gas diffuses into the extended extravascular region, bounded by *b.* The radial diffusion equation is given by,

$$D \frac{\partial^2 p}{\partial r^2} + \frac{D}{r} \frac{\partial p}{\partial r} = \frac{\partial p}{\partial t} , \tag{C-1}$$

with the tissue tensions, p, equal to the venous tensions, p_v, at the vascular interfaces, a and b. The solution to the tissue diffusion equation is given in Appendix B,

$$p - p_v = (p_i - p_v) \frac{4}{(b/2)^2 - a^2} \sum_{n=1}^{\infty} \frac{1}{\epsilon_n^2} \frac{J_1^2(\epsilon_n b/2)}{J_0^2(\epsilon_n a) - J_1(\epsilon_n b/2)} \exp(-\epsilon_n^2 Dt) , \tag{C-2}$$

with ϵ_n eigenvalue roots of the boundary conditions,

$$J_0(\epsilon_n a) Y_1(\epsilon_n b/2) - Y_0(\epsilon_n a) J_1(\epsilon_n b/2) = 0 , \tag{C-3}$$

for J and Y Bessel and Neumann functions, order 1 and 0. Perfusion limiting is applied as a boundary condition through the venous tension, p_v, by enforcing a mass balance across both the vascular and cellular regions at a,

$$\frac{\partial p_v}{\partial t} = -\kappa(p_v - p_a) - \frac{3}{a} S_p D \left[\frac{\partial p}{\partial r} \right]_{r=a} , \tag{C-3}$$

with S_p the ratio of cellular to blood gas solubilities, κ the perfusion constant, and p_a the arterial tension. The coupled set relate tension, gas flow, diffusion and perfusion, and solubility in a complex feedback loop.

The thermodynamic trigger point for decompression sickness is the volume fraction, χ, of separated gas, coupled to mass balance. Denoting the separated gas partial pressure, P_{N_2}, under worse case conditions of zero gas elimination upon decompression, the separated gas fraction is estimated,

$$\chi P_{N_2} = S_c (p - P_{N_2}) , \tag{C-4}$$

with S_c the cellular gas solubility. The separated nitrogen partial pressure, P_{N_2} is taken up by the inherent unsaturation, and given by (*fsw*),

$$P_{N_2} = P + 3.21 , \tag{C-5}$$

in the original Hills formulation, but other estimates have been employed. Mechanical fluid injection pain, depending on the injection pressure, δ, can be related to the separated gas fraction, χ, through the tissue modulus, K,

$$K\chi = \delta \,, \tag{C-6}$$

so that a decompression criteria requires,

$$K\chi \leq \delta \,, \tag{C-7}$$

with δ in the range, for $K = 3.7 \times 10^4$ *dyne cm*$^{-2}$,

$$0.34 \leq \delta \leq 1.13 \; fsw \,.$$

Identification of the separated phase volume as a critical indicator is a significant development in decompression theory.

APPENDIX D: VARYING PERMEABILITY MODEL

The critical bubble radius, r_0, at fixed pressure, P_0, represents the cutoff for growth upon decompression to lessure pressure. Nuclei larger than r_0 are thought to grow upon decompression. Additionally, following an initial compression, $\Delta P = P - P_0$, a smaller class of micronuclei of critical radius, r can be excited into growth with decompression. If r_0 is the critical radius at P_0, then the smaller family, r, excited by decompression from P, obeys,

$$\frac{1}{r} = \frac{1}{r_0} + \frac{\Delta P}{158} \,, \tag{D-1}$$

with ΔP measured in *fsw*, and r in *microns.* Table 3 lists critical radii, r, excited by sea-level compressions ($P_0 = 33$ *fsw*), assuming $r_0 = .8$ *microns.* Entries also represent the equilibrium critical radius at pressure, P.

The permissible gradient, G, is written for each compartment, τ, using the standard formalism,

$$G = G_0 + \Delta G \, d \,, \tag{D-2}$$

at depth $d = P - 33$ *fsw.* A non-stop bounce exposure, followed by direct return to the surface, thus allows G_0 for that compartment. Both G_0 and ΔG are tabulated in Table 5b, with ΔG suggested by Buhlmann and Workman.

excitation, G^{min}, initially probing r, and taking into account regeneration of nuclei over time scales τ_r, is *(fsw),*

$$G^{min} = \frac{2\gamma\,(\gamma_c - \gamma)}{\gamma_c\, r(t)} = \frac{11.01}{r(t)}\ , \tag{D-3}$$

with,

$$r\,(t) = r + (r_0 - r)\,[1 - exp\,(-\lambda_r t)], \tag{D-4}$$

γ, γ_c film, surfactant surface tensions, that is, $\gamma = 17.9$ *dyne/cm,* $\gamma_c = 257$ *dyne/cm,* and λ_r the inverse of the regeneration time for stabilized gas micronuclei (many days). Prolonged exposure leads to saturation, and the largest permissible gradient, G^{sat}, takes the form *(fsw)*, in all compartments.

$$G^{sat} = \frac{58.6}{r} - 49.9 = .372\,P + 11.01\ . \tag{D-5}$$

On the other hand, G^{min} is the excitation threshold, the amount by which the surrounding tension must exceed internal bubble pressure to just support growth.

Although the actual size distribution of gas nuclei in humans in unknown, experiments *in vitro* suggest that a decaying exponential is reasonable,

$$n = N\ exp\,(-\beta r), \tag{D-6}$$

with β a constant, and N a convenient normalization factor across the distribution. For small values of the argument, βr,

$$exp\,(-\ \beta r) \approx 1 - \beta r\ , \tag{D-7}$$

as a nice simplification. For a stabilized distribution, n_0, accommodated by the body at fixed pressure, P_0, the excess number of nuclei, Δn, excited by compression-decompression from new pressure, P, is,

$$\Delta n = n_0 - \mathrm{n} \approx \mathrm{N}\,\beta r_0\left[1 - \frac{r}{r_0}\right]\ . \tag{D-8}$$

For large compressions-decompression, Δn is large, while for small compressions-decompression, Δn is small. When Δn is folded over the gradient, G, in time, the product serves as a critical volume indicator and can be used as a limit point in the following way.

The rate at which gas inflates in tissue depends upon both the excess bubble number, Δn, and the gradient, G. The critical volume hypothesis requires that the integral of the product of the two must always remain less than some limit point, $\alpha\ V^{crit}$, with α proportionality constant,

$$\int_0^\infty \Delta n\, G\, dt = \alpha\, V^{crit}, \tag{D-9}$$

for V^{crit} the limiting gas volume. Assuming that gradients are constant during decompression, t_d, while decaying exponentially to zero afterwards, and taking the limiting condition of the equal sign, yields simply for a bounce dive,

$$\Delta n\ G\ (t_d + \lambda^{-1}) = \alpha V^{crit}. \tag{D-10}$$

In terms of earlier parameters, one more constant, δ, closes the set defined by,

$$\delta = \frac{\gamma_c\, \alpha\, V^{crit}}{\gamma \beta r_0 N} = 7180\ fsw\ \text{min}, \tag{D-11}$$

so that,

$$\left[1 - \frac{r}{r_0}\right] G\,(t_d + \lambda^{-1}) = \delta\ \frac{\gamma}{\gamma_c} = 500.8\ fsw\ \text{min}. \tag{D-12}$$

The five parameters, γ, γ_c, δ, λ_r r_0, are five of the six fundamental constants in the varying permeability model. The remaining parameter, λ_m, interpolating bounce and saturation exposures, represents the inverse time constant modulating multi-diving. Bubble growth experiments suggest that λ_m^{-1} is in the neighborhood of an hour.

The depth at which a compartment controls an exposure, and the excitation radius as a function of half-life, τ, in the range, $12 \leq d \leq 220\ fsw$, satisfy,

$$\frac{r}{r_0} = .9 - .43\ exp\,(-\ \lambda_h\, \tau) \tag{D-13}$$

with $\lambda_h = .0559\ \text{min}^{-1}$. The regeneration constant, λ_r, is on the order of inverse days, that is, $\lambda_r = 0.495\ days^{-1}$. Characteristic half-times, τ_r and τ_h, take the values $\tau_r = 14\ days$ and $\tau_h = 12.4$ min. For large τ, r is close to r_0, while for small τ, r is on the order of $.5\ r_0$. At sea level, $r_0 = .8\ microns$ as discussed.

APPENDIX E: REDUCED GRADIENT BUBBLE MODEL

The phase integral for multi-exposures is written,

$$\sum_{j=1}^{J} \left[\Delta n\, G\, t_{d_j} + \int_0^{t_j} \Delta n\, G\, dt \right] \leq \alpha\, V^{crit}, \quad \text{(E-1)}$$

with the index j denoting each dive segment, up to a total of J, and t_j the surface interval after the jth segment. For the inequality to hold, that is, for the sum of all growth rate items to total less than $\alpha\ V^{crit}$, obviously each term must be less than the $\alpha\ V^{crit}$. Assuming that $t_j \longrightarrow \infty$, gives,

$$\sum_{j=1}^{J-1} \left[\Delta n\, G\, [t_{d_j} + \lambda^{-1} - \lambda^{-1}\, exp(-\lambda t_j)] \right] + \Delta n\, G\, (t_{d_j} + \lambda^{-1}) \leq \alpha\, V^{crit}. \quad \text{(E-2)}$$

Defining G_j,

$$\Delta n\ G_j(t_{d_j} + \lambda^{-1}) = \Delta n\ G\ (t_{d_j} + \lambda^{-1}) - \Delta n\ G\lambda^{-1}\ exp\,(-\lambda t_{j-1}), \quad \text{(E-3)}$$

for $j = 2$ to J, and,

$$\Delta n\ G_1 = \Delta n\ G\,, \quad \text{(E-4)}$$

for $j = 1$, it follows that

$$\sum_{j=1}^{J} \Delta n\ G_j\ (t_{d_j} + \lambda^{-1}) \leq \alpha\ V^{crit}, \quad \text{(E-5)}$$

with the important property,

$$G_j \leq G\,. \quad \text{(E-6)}$$

This implies we employ reduced repetitive gradients extracted from bounce gradients by writing,

$$G_j = \xi_j\, G\,, \quad \text{(E-7)}$$

with ξ_j a *multi-diving* fraction requisitely satisfying,

$$0 \leq \xi_j \leq 1\,, \quad \text{(E-8)}$$

so that, as needed,

$$\Delta n\ G_j \leq \Delta n\ G\ . \tag{E-9}$$

The fractions, ξ, applied to G always reduce them.

As time and repetitive frequency increase, the body's ability to eliminate excess bubbles and nuclei decreases, so that we restrict the permissible bubble excess in time by writing,

$$\Delta n(t_{j-1}^{cum}) = N\beta r_0 \left[1 - \frac{r(t_{j-1}^{cum})}{r_0} \right] = \Delta n\ exp(-\lambda_r t_{j-1}^{cum})\ ,$$

$$t_{j-1}^{cum} = \sum_{i=1}^{j-1} t_i\ , \tag{E-10}$$

with t_{j-1}^{cum} cumulative surface interval time. A reduction factor, η_j^{reg}, accounting for creation of new micronuclei is taken to be the ratio of present excess over initial excess, written,

$$\eta_j^{reg} = \frac{\Delta n(t_{j-1}^{cum})}{\Delta n} = exp(-\lambda_r t_{j-1}^{cum})\ . \tag{E-11}$$

For deeper-than-previous diving, the gradient is restricted by the ratio (minimum value) of the bubble excess on the present segment to the bubble excess at the deepest point over segments. The gradient reduction, η_j^{exc}, is then written,

$$\eta_j^{exc} = \frac{(\Delta n)_{\max}}{(\Delta n)_j} = \frac{(rd)_{\max}}{(rd)_j}\ , \tag{E-12}$$

with *rd* the product of the appropriate excitation radius and depth. Because bubble elimination periods are shortened over repetitive dives, compared to intervals for bounce dives, the gradient reduction, η_j^{rep}, is proportional to the difference between maximum and actual surface bubble inflation rate, that is,

$$\eta_j^{rep} = 1 - \left[1 - \frac{G^{min}}{G} \right] exp(-\lambda_m t_{j-1})\ , \tag{E-13}$$

with t_{j-1} consecutive surface interval time, λ_m^{-1} on the order of an hour, and G^{min} the smallest G_0 in Table 5b or the mechanical surface tension pressure of characteristic bubbles.

Finally, for multi-diving, the gradient reduction factor, ξ, is defined by the product of the three η,

$$\xi_j = \eta_j^{exc}\,\eta_j^{rep}\,\eta_j^{reg} = \frac{(\Delta n)_{max}}{(\Delta n)_j}\left[1 - \left[1 - \frac{G^{min}}{G}\right] exp\,(-\lambda_m t_{j-1})\right] exp\,(-\lambda_r t_{j-1}^{cum})\;, \tag{E-14}$$

with t_{j-1} consecutive interval time, and t_{j-1}^{cum} cumulative interval time, as noted. Since bubble numbers increase with depth, reduction in permissible gradient is commensurate. Multi-day diving is mostly impacted by λ_r, while repetitive diving mostly by λ_m. Obviously, the critical tension, M, takes the form,

$$M = \xi\,(G_0 + \Delta G\, d) + P\,. \tag{E-15}$$

APPENDIX F: PROBABILITY AND MAXIMUM LIKELIHOOD

The measure of any random occurrence, ρ, can be a complicated function of many parameters, $q = (q_1, q_2, \ldots q_\kappa)$, with the only constraint,

$$0 \leq \rho(q) \leq 1\;, \tag{F-1}$$

for appropriate values of q. The measure of nonoccurrence, σ, is then by conservation of probability,

$$\sigma(q) = 1 - \rho(q)\;, \tag{F-2}$$

over the same range of q, with,

$$0 \leq \sigma(q) \leq 1\;. \tag{F-3}$$

Multi-valued functions, $\rho(q_1, q_2, \ldots q_K)$ are often constructed, with specific form dictated by theory or observation over many trials. In decompression applications, the parameters, q, may well be the bubble-nucleation rate, number of venous gas emboli, degree of supersaturation, amount of pressure reduction, volume of separated gas, ascent rate, or combinations thereof. Parameters may be also integrated over time in any sequence of events, though such measures are more difficult to analyze over arbitrary trial numbers.

The likelihood of any outcome, Φ, of N trials is a product of the individual measures of the form,

$$\Phi(n) = \rho^n (1 - \rho)^m = \rho^n \sigma^m\;, \tag{F-4}$$

given n failures and m successes (n cases of decompression sickness, and m cases without decompression sickness), with,

$$n + m = N . \tag{F-5}$$

The logarithm of the likelihood, Ψ, is easier to use in calculations and takes the form,

$$\Psi(n) = ln\ \Phi(n) = n\ ln\ \rho + m\ ln\ (1 - \rho) , \tag{F-6}$$

and is maximized,

$$\frac{\partial \Psi}{\partial \rho} = 0 , \tag{F-7}$$

when, for appropriate values of n, m, and ρ,

$$\frac{n}{\rho} - \frac{m}{1 - \rho} = 0 . \tag{F-8}$$

Almost trivially, this requires,

$$\rho = \frac{n}{n + m} = \frac{n}{N} ,$$

$$\sigma = 1 - \rho = \frac{m}{n + m} = \frac{m}{N} , \tag{F-9}$$

Thus the likelihood function is maximized when the failure measure, ρ, is the ratio of actual failures to trials, and similarly in the case of successes. For multi-valued probability functions, $\rho(q_1, q_2, \ldots q_K)$, the maximization generalizes,

$$\frac{\partial \Psi}{\partial \rho} = \sum_{i=1}^{K} \frac{\partial \Psi}{\partial q_i} \frac{\partial q_i}{\partial \rho} = 0 , \tag{F-10}$$

satisfied when,

$$\frac{\partial \Psi}{\partial q_i} = 0\ (i = 1, K) . \tag{F-11}$$

The above set can be solved by analytical or numerical methods on a computer.

Decompression phenomena are characterized by binary statistics, equivalently binomial probability. Binomial distribution functions permit calculation of exact probabilities of any set of binary occurrences. The probability, Π, of a random sample of size, N, with n occurrences of decompression sickness and m nonoccurrences, is given by,

$$\Pi(n) = \frac{N!}{n!m!} \rho^m \sigma^n \frac{N!}{n!m!} \Phi(n) , \qquad \text{(F-12)}$$

with ρ the underlying incidence. The probability of no decompression sickness in any set of N trials is simply,

$$\Pi(0) = \sigma^N = \Phi(0) , \qquad \text{(F-13)}$$

while the probability of all cases of decompression sickness in N trials is similarly,

$$\Pi(N) = \rho^N = \Phi(N) . \qquad \text{(F-14)}$$

The discrete probability distribution is normalized to one, that is,

$$\sum_{n=0}^{N} \Pi(n) = 1 , \qquad \text{(F-15)}$$

so that the cumulative probability for more than n cases of decompression sickness, $\Pi_>(n)$,

$$\Pi_>(n) = \sum_{j=n+1}^{N} \Pi(j) = 1 - \sum_{j=0}^{n} \Pi(j) , \qquad \text{(F-16)}$$

and the probability of less than n cases of decompression sickness, $\Pi_<(n)$, is similarly,

$$\Pi_<(n) = \sum_{j=0}^{n-1} \Pi(j) = 1 - \sum_{j=n}^{N} \Pi(j) . \qquad \text{(F-17)}$$

For instance, if we assume 10 trial dives, with an underlying incidence of .05, quite simply the individual probabilities are given by,

$$P(0) = .95^{10} = .60 ,$$

$$P(10) = .05^{10} = 10^{-13} ,$$

while the cumulative probabilities are,

$$\Pi_{>}(0) = 1 - .60 = .40 ,$$

$$\Pi_{<}(0) = 1 - 1 = 0 ,$$

$$\Pi_{>}(10) = 1 - 1 = 0 ,$$

$$\Pi_{<}(10) = 1 - 10^{-13}.$$

In dealing with a large number of decompression procedures spanning a significant range in depth, time, and environmental factors, an integrated approach to maximum likelihood and risk is needed. Integral measures, $\rho(t)$ and $\sigma(t)$, might be defined over the decompression risk, ζ,

$$\rho(t) = 1 - exp \left[- \int_0^t \zeta(t') \, dt' \right] ,$$

$$\sigma(t) = exp \left[- \int_0^t \zeta(t') \, dt' \right] , \qquad \text{(F-18)}$$

with t' any convenient time scale. The function, ζ, is any artibtrary instantaneous measure of decompression risk. Using Eq. (F-18) in the likelihood function, and then maximizing according to the data, permits the estimation of all risk constants in ζ.

As an example of the maximum likelihood method, consider the general case of a simple probability model applied to the test data, that is, assume that the risk, ζ, is an exponentially decreasing function of time, with q a constant,

$$\zeta(t') = exp\,(-qt') , \qquad \text{(F-19)}$$

and that we track risk over all time, $0 \le t \le \infty$. Then,

$$\rho(\infty) = 1 - exp\,(-q^{-1}) ,$$

$$\sigma(\infty) = exp\,(-q^{-1}) . \qquad \text{(F-20)}$$

Suppose in applying this risk criteria to 10 dives, 2 cases of decompression sickness are observed, and thus 8 cases without decompression sickness. Accordingly, the likelihood logarithm takes the form, with $n = 2$ and $m = 8$,

$$\Psi = ln\,[1 - exp\,(-q^{-1})] + ln\,[exp\,(-q^{-1})], \tag{F-21}$$

maximized,

$$\frac{\partial \Psi}{\partial q} = 0\,, \tag{F-22}$$

when,

$$1 - exp\,(-q^{-1}) = .2\,,$$

$$exp\,(-q^{-1}) = .8\,, \tag{F-23}$$

from which,

$$\frac{1}{q} = -\,ln\,(.8)\,. \tag{F-24}$$